Praise for *Cancer Confidential*

"Touching. Deep. Powerful."
Nancy Beal, Communications Consultant and Author of *Alex Tilley: An Endurable Legacy*

"The author and I share many things in common, but I was deeply touched by his acute sensitivity to the emotional dramas of oncology, which arose not just from his acting training but also from his experience with close family cancer and death. Fascinating insights as roles are reversed and emotion takes its place in the drama of life – and death."
Lord Michael Cashman, Member of the House of Lords of the United Kingdom and Author of *One of Them*

"All the [medical] world's a stage! In elegant prose, with Felliniesque flights into whimsical metaphor, physician-historian-playwright Charles Hayter describes his encounters with cancer, as a doctor and as a son, and how the experience changed him as a person. Sensitive to the arrogance and obfuscation of his clinical colleagues, he advocates for the underappreciated power of radiation therapy in cancer care and for truth in all relationships."
Jacalyn M. Duffin, Professor Emerita and Hannah Chair of the History of Medicine, Queen's University

"There are many books written by surgeons and physicians about their life in medicine, but none are like this one. Most are faintly veiled tales of personal heroics, or writings about the wonders of medicine, but this book stands out as a personal story that is honest and sometimes raw, of patient challenges and loss, and an informative story of the place of radiation in modern cancer care. Charles Hayter is open about the personal pain in his family relationships, his distressing tensions with both mother and father, and his eventual recognition and revealing of his gay life. He could have told the

story of radiation oncology and cancer patients without revealing himself, but that honesty is one of the powerful appeals of this wonderful book."
Jock Murray, OC, ONS, MD, FRCPC, MACP, Dean Emeritus and Professor of Medicine, Dalhousie University

Cancer
Confidential

Backstage
Dramas
in the
Radiation
Clinic

Charles Hayter, MD

ÆVO UTP

Aevo UTP
An imprint of University of Toronto Press
Toronto Buffalo London
utorontopress.com

Library and Archives Canada Cataloguing in Publication

Title: Cancer confidential : backstage dramas in the radiation clinic /
    Charles Hayter, MD.
Names: Hayter, Charles, author.
Identifiers: Canadiana (print) 20220211132 | Canadiana (ebook) 20220211248 |
    ISBN 9781487528157 (cloth) | ISBN 9781487528171 (EPUB) |
    ISBN 9781487528164 (PDF)
Subjects: LCSH: Cancer – Patients. | LCSH: Cancer – Patients – Family relationships. |
    LCSH: Cancer – Psychological aspects. | LCSH: Cancer – Patients – Death. |
    LCSH: Cancer – Radiotherapy.
Classification: LCC RC263 .H39 2022 | DDC 616.99/4 – dc23

ISBN 978-1-4875-2815-7 (cloth)   ISBN 978-1-4875-2817-1 (EPUB)
                                 ISBN 978-1-4875-2816-4 (PDF)

Printed in Canada

We wish to acknowledge the land on which the University of Toronto Press operates. This land is
the traditional territory of the Wendat, the Anishnaabeg, the Haudenosaunee, the Métis, and the
Mississaugas of the Credit First Nation.

University of Toronto Press acknowledges the financial support of the Government of Canada,
the Canada Council for the Arts, and the Ontario Arts Council, an agency of the Government of
Ontario, for its publishing activities.

Canada Council **Conseil des Arts**
for the Arts **du Canada**

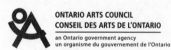

ONTARIO ARTS COUNCIL
CONSEIL DES ARTS DE L'ONTARIO
an Ontario government agency
un organisme du gouvernement de l'Ontario

Funded by the   Financé par le
Government   gouvernement
of Canada   du Canada

Canadä

MIX
Paper from
responsible sources
FSC FSC® C016245

For cancer patients and their families everywhere,
in the hope they may never feel alone

Contents

Disclaimer

This book describes encounters with patients and families inspired by incidents that occurred during my career as a radiation oncologist. I have taken care to protect the original patients' confidences by altering details of gender, ethnicity, occupation, and personal relationships. In fact, the characters of this book are more fictional composites of persons sharing similar characteristics than representations of specific individuals. Because cancer is such a common disease, readers will inevitably find similarities to their own circumstances, but such similarities are purely coincidental. In addition, my depictions of medical colleagues are fictions inspired by characteristics of individuals encountered during my career.

I have woven the story of my father's cancer through the stories of patients and their families. The events of my father's illness took place more than thirty years ago, and my memory for the facts sometimes failed me. I have filled some gaps by consulting my journals, letters from my mother, and conversations with my siblings and children. I confess I have had to fill other gaps with conjecture. However, I have striven to be faithful to the emotional truth of what happened. Like other memoirists, I can often recall the emotion better than the facts.

Finally, this book also contains descriptions of medical treatments and procedures. Because this book is part memoir, some of them are outdated. No description of a treatment in this book should be taken as a recommendation, and patients should always consult with their own physicians before embarking on treatment.

Prologue: Medicine as Theatre

The summer between my second and third years of medical school proved to be momentous. Not only was my second child, a son, born, but I undertook a summer internship in the field that later became my career: radiation oncology. In the evening, my newborn son's writhings and happy gurgles were an effective antidote to the often grim daytime experience in the cancer centre.

At thirty – older than many of my classmates – I had taken a circuitous path to medical school, having first pursued an undergraduate degree in English and drama, a graduate degree in drama, two years of teaching drama, and crash courses in the basic sciences needed to enter medicine.

When I entered the gritty world of medicine, I thought I'd left the make-believe world of theatre far behind. One morning that summer, garbed in the crisp white jacket of a medical student, I sat in the busy workroom behind the examining rooms, waiting to follow my professor into a room to see a patient. As I observed the doctors preparing to see their patients, a frisson of familiarity swept over me. Of course! It was just like being in the green room backstage at a theatre. Just as actors make last-minute adjustments to their costumes or makeup before they step on stage, so I spotted doctors straightening their ties or smoothing their hair just before they stepped into the examining rooms. They skimmed through patients' files to remind themselves of facts just as actors quickly flip through their scripts to refresh their lines. They consulted treatment

xii   Prologue: Medicine as Theatre

algorithms pinned to the walls like the prompt sheets pinned to the timbers of an Elizabethan theatre. I overheard them referring to their patients not by name but by "stage" as if they were naming a character. It wasn't "I'm going to see Mary Brown," it was "I'm going to see a T3 breast cancer."

My professor that day was a senior radiation oncologist, a short, white-haired man whose gentle, soft-spoken demeanour reminded me of my maternal grandfather. After he scanned his patient's chart, he frowned at me over the top of his wire-rimmed glasses.

"This is going to be difficult," he murmured.

Without further explanation, he dusted his lapels, smoothed a few stray wisps, opened the examining room door, and stepped inside. Wondering what he meant, I trotted behind him.

Inside, a middle-aged man and woman sat huddled together as if bracing for bad news. The man's face was craggy and grey, his wife's corrugated in anxiety.

"Doctor. I hope you have good news for us," the woman blurted.

The professor sat down, paused, and leaned towards them. "I'm afraid it's not. Your X-rays show the lung cancer has grown."

The woman emitted a gasp and drew her husband close. He dropped his gaze to the floor. For a moment there was no sound except for the woman's whimpers and the man's raspy wheeze. Finally, the man looked up and glared at the doctor. "Why the hell did you put me through that goddamn radiation?" His voice cracked with anger.

"What now? Are you just going to let him die?" his wife said in a high-pitched quaver.

Emotion flooded the space. It felt like the walls of the tiny, cramped examining room were about to blow open. I'd never experienced anything like it before. I felt a strong urge to bolt.

Over the next few minutes, I watched in wonder and admiration as the professor defused the situation, not so much through his words, but through his vocal tone and body language. As he explained in soft tones what might lie ahead, he maintained steady eye contact, nodded reassuringly, and occasionally rested his hand on the wife's arm. His physical gestures inspired comfort and hope in a dire situation. By the end of the session, the couple had visibly relaxed – and so had I.

His behaviour contrasted with that of another doctor I'd seen on a different day. She remained standing while delivering bad news in the direct, staccato style of a TV anchor, then wheeled and abruptly left the room, leaving her patient – and me – noticeably even more distressed than at the beginning.

The behaviour of these doctors struck another chord: it reminded me of the way actors manipulate their voices and bodies to provoke emotional reactions in the audience. It was performance, pure and simple – performance supported by the familiar costumes and props of medicine: white coats, stethoscopes, and other technical accoutrements. Aristotle described the goal of theatre as *catharsis*, the emotional release from sadness or joy experienced at the denouement of a play. As anyone who's ever been surprised to find themselves blubbering uncontrollably at the conclusion of a movie or play can attest, catharsis is a real phenomenon. Just as a play induces catharsis in the audience, so the doctors' performances elicited powerful emotional responses in their patients.

As my medical career progressed, I often felt I was back in the theatre. Learning to be a doctor, and later an oncologist, was just like learning a role in a play: I had to assume a particular deportment and vocabulary, and learn how to wear the costumes and use the props with authority and confidence. As I'd already noticed, in the theatre of medicine patients became characters identified not by their real names but by diagnosis or stage. My inner humanist bucked against this reductionism, but as time went on I picked it up. During ward rounds, I found myself saying to a nurse, "Boy, that T4 gastric cancer over there looks anemic" or "That T3 oesophagus in Room 348 needs a feeding tube." I was masking the patient's identity, and also protecting myself with a tough goalie mask that deflected painful shots from a suffering human.

I discovered that "performance" is part of the *lingua franca* of oncology. In the late 1940s, Dr. David Karnofsky, a pioneering American medical oncologist, devised a scale to measure the ability of a patient to withstand chemotherapy that became known as the Karnofsky Performance Status Scale (KPS). The scale rated a patient's "performance" in increments from 100 per cent (complete well-being) to 0 per cent (death). It was a convenient way of reducing a whole host of complex physical and psychological factors to a number on a scale. A score of 40 per cent, for example, indicated disability requiring special care or assistance. The KPS quickly became a routine part of my medical vocabulary. I became as adept at labelling patients by "performance" as by stage, and the patient's "performance" became their ticket to treatment – only patients with good performances were allowed entry to the rigorous world of chemotherapy or radiation. But like all auditions, it was highly subjective: it didn't take into account the biases of the auditioner or day-to-day fluctuation in a patient's condition, or the host of physical and social factors that might cause these changes.

If doctors and patients are dramatic figures, what story are they enacting? Cancer patients' obituaries frequently refer to their experience as a "journey" or a "battle." Like all clichés, these terms carry an element of truth. Cancer patients' journeys often follow the three-act structure that underpins traditional dramatic writing from fairy tales to TV series to grand operas: the hero presented with a challenge, the hero experiencing trials and battles of increasing difficulty, perhaps aided by a friend or mentor, and the hero's transformation as a result of the experience. The transformation may involve a return home or self-actualization towards a new path. The cancer diagnosis is the challenge or call to action that prompts a quest for healing. Patients depart their ordinary lives and enter the dark, unfamiliar world of the cancer centre with its mysterious implements and potions. Here, they meet a mentor – the oncologist – who guides them through this unknown, terrifying land and attempts to cure them. Rid of disease, but sometimes not, patients eventually return to their ordinary lives. Like the archetypal heroes of drama, they are profoundly changed by their experiences. Many cancer survivors have described the deep spiritual effect of a life-threatening illness that encourages them to make course corrections in their lives.

Doctors, too, work through their own three acts: Diagnosis, Treatment, and Outcome. In Act One, we make a diagnosis. In Act Two, we administer treatments, often of increasing intensity, that result in success or failure to cure. In the final act, the patient is discharged home, either fully recovered or to die. This paradigm is first inculcated in medical school and later becomes an unconscious part of our thinking and attitude towards our patients. Make a diagnosis, apply a remedy, and either cure or fail to cure the patient.

These acts are embedded in the scripts that guide cancer treatment. Perhaps more than any other field of medicine, oncology is driven by protocols: summaries, often in algorithmic form, of the diagnostic and therapeutic steps in the "management" of patients with a particular form of cancer. Go into that backstage area of a cancer clinic, and you'll soon encounter protocol sheets pinned to the board or shimmering on the phones or tablets of the doctors for easy reference. You'll overhear doctors asking each other "What's the protocol for X cancer?" or "How do I manage cancer of the Y?" In case conferences, disputes are frequently resolved by reference to the holy book of a protocol. Much of my time as a resident was spent studying and memorizing protocols, in preparation for examination questions such as "Describe the management of cancer of the X."

Treatment protocols serve important purposes. For one thing, they ensure thoroughness of care. Oncologists are fallible, and a particular scan useful in staging might get missed if not for the reminder on the protocol. Despite decades of research on cancer, there remain many uncertainties about the best treatments, and a protocol is a consensus summary of the current best approach based on available evidence. It ensures patients with the same cancer receive consistent, up-to-date "management." For a trainee, treatment protocols are a convenient way of organizing knowledge.

But these scripts have serious deficiencies. First, protocols miscast doctors in the role of Hero. Patients have little if any agency in the drama. They are mere puppets whose diseases – indeed, lives – are to be "managed." Doctors don't see themselves in their true role, which is mentor or guide. This mismatch between doctors' and patients' expectation of their roles underlies many of the ethical and interpersonal conflicts that occur in medicine.

Second, and more important, they do not address the emotional and psychological needs of patients and their families. I entered oncology practice brimming with enthusiasm to apply the protocols I'd learned to my patients, but I quickly and painfully discovered a host of unexpected traps, pitfalls, snares, and hidden dangers lay in my way – dangers not described in the protocols. Because I had mistakenly adopted the Hero's role, with its attendant hubris, I was often unaware of the obstacles ahead and blindsided when things didn't go as expected.

Some of these obstacles came from patients: their unwillingness, sometimes outright refusal, to follow the script. Some of them even chose their own, independent path. Others were content to follow my advice, but demanded special attention. Other obstacles came from family members, such as children who interfered in the medical treatment of their parents. I saw how a cancer diagnosis can fracture families, pushing their members apart instead of closer. Still other obstacles came from colleagues, especially surgeons, often unwilling to give patients choices between surgery and non-operative approaches such as radiation. For patients, families, and colleagues alike, my work was frequently stymied by the curtain of silence drawn around cancer that prevented open communication.

I also faced internal obstacles. I hadn't foreseen the extent to which medical knowledge is limited and the number of times when the path is unclear. My own doubts about which path to follow often led to hesitancy of decision. I hadn't anticipated failure, both to cure and to avoid complications, and its attendant disappointment and guilt. I wasn't prepared for the overpowering displays of emotion by patients and families that sometimes left me fearful, cowering, and tempted to make inappropriate decisions. I hadn't recognized my own unwillingness to utter the truth in some uncomfortable situations. Many cancer journeys have unhappy endings, and I wasn't adequately prepared for the daily onslaught of breaking bad news.

The technical treatment of cancer, such as aiming radiation beams, was easy compared to navigating the terrain of these emotional minefields. As my career unfolded, many of these situations occurred so repeatedly as to form recognizable motifs with central characters who appeared with such regularity they can be regarded as archetypes: the Reticent Doctor who never uses the word cancer, the Interfering Child who sabotages a treatment plan, the Bossy Patient who demands to go to the head of the queue, the Confused Patient whose concerns echo my inner uncertainties, or the Shunned Patient who comes to me as a last resort.

As I stood downstage with my patient, trying valiantly to stick to the script, I was always aware one or more of these figures lay waiting in the wings, ready to leap onto the stage, disrupt my performance, and steal the show with their diva antics, which often involved denial, avoidance, or conflict. These characters did not appear in the Dramatis Personae of any script I'd learned. Like my colleagues, I felt unequipped to deal with them. I'd witnessed colleagues throw temper tantrums at the thwarting of their "management plans." I too felt confused, angry, and frustrated when things didn't go according to the script. I often foisted the management of these disrupters onto my nursing or social work colleagues.

My goal in this book is to drag these characters and their dramas from the wings to the glare of the footlights, where they can be examined more closely, and their subtext, the complex, powerful, and often irrational undercurrent of emotions, can be revealed. The dramas can be understood for what they are: manifestations of primal human emotions such as fear, desperation, anxiety, and anger aroused by a diagnosis of cancer. In the glare of the downstage light, they lose their power and can be acknowledged as recurring, predictable aspects of the drama.

The chapters that follow depict a series of the most common scenarios from my thirty-year practice in radiation oncology. If I, as one oncologist, have encountered these situations frequently enough to recognize patterns, I assume other patients and colleagues have met with them regularly too and will find points of recognition with their own experience. My hope is that this recognition will empower cancer patients and those who care about them to face their own situations with insight, grace, and compassion.

The grand *mise en scene* for the scenarios is the specialty of radiation oncology. In each chapter, I've painted this backdrop in some detail – including its history and applications – because, despite its widespread use and long history, it remains so poorly understood. Over my long career as a radiation oncologist I've been reminded almost daily of the misconceptions surrounding the field. Patients come to me frightened of radiation "burns," when it doesn't work by burning. Or they wonder why their cancers haven't disappeared overnight, when it can take days or even weeks to see a response. Worse of all, they view it as a remedy of last resort: If they're sending me for radiation, they've given up, I must be dying!

These misconceptions are reinforced by popular media that often depict radiation therapy as a barbaric process, something out of B-grade sci-fi movies involving ray-cannons shooting painful lightning bolts. Sadly too, they are reinforced in the writings of some of the leading physician-authors of our day. Paul Kalanithi's 2016 best-seller *When Breath Becomes Air* is an account of a surgeon's personal experience of lung cancer. As I turned its pages, deeply moved by his account of months of wracking, unremitting back pain caused by cancer, I waited for a referral for palliative radiation, which might have relieved his pain and allowed him to reduce his painkillers, but it never came. Siddhartha Mukherjee's Pulitzer-prize winning "biography of cancer," *The Emperor of All Maladies*, gives short shrift to radiotherapy and perpetuates the burning myth by using verbs such as "scald."

My sensitivity to the hidden emotional dramas of oncology arose not just from my drama training, but also from my experience with my father's cancer and death. Shortly after I graduated as a radiation oncologist, my father was diagnosed with terminal prostate cancer. My medical training had not prepared me for the difficult personal journey ahead, which involved a host of unpredictable and often unwelcome feelings and thoughts. My experience with his illness laid the groundwork for my observations of how individuals and families deal with cancer. In my practice, I witnessed many of the same responses and behaviours I'd experienced on a personal level during his illness. My personal story of my father's illness provides a frame for the individual patient scenarios described in this book.

It began on a crisp autumn day in Calgary, Alberta, in 1989.

1

The Medical Son

In 1989, as I creep from the wings onto the medical stage, my father, Russell, sixty-four, is about to exit from a long career as a specialist in physical medicine and rehabilitation. He lives with my mother, Joyce, in a ranch-style bungalow in a sprawling suburb of Calgary, Alberta. On a clear day, you can make out the glint of the peaks of the Rockies beyond the green, rolling foothills surrounding the city.

The only other occupant of the bungalow is their beagle, Trixie. After my parents' move to Calgary a decade earlier, my younger sister, Sally, remained in Winnipeg, my family's landing place in Canada after its emigration from England in 1963. My brother, Robert, ten years my junior, has returned to England, where his marriage to an English woman in the spring of 1989 was to be the final joyous family gathering for my parents. Like many couples at this juncture of life, my parents eagerly anticipate many years of retirement.

In late September, after attending a medical conference in Edmonton, I travel south to Calgary to pay a brief visit to my parents before heading back east to my home, at that time in New Brunswick. On the morning after my arrival, I stand alone in their kitchen, gazing through the window, marvelling at how my father has transformed an arid patch of dusty prairie, where not long ago buffalo hooves pounded, into a replica of a perfect English garden. There's a rectangle of manicured lawn, its surface smooth and pristine as a bowling green, edged by beds of flowers, arrayed from front to back by height. Touched by early frosts, the fading, crumpled blooms sag and tilt like rows of broad Edwardian hats on mourners at a funeral. My father was born and raised in colonial India, in the waning days of the British Empire. For him there is nothing unusual about colonizing soil with foreign plants.

Now, he comes into view, a tall, handsome man with a broad forehead surmounted by neatly combed thick black hair, rendered to gleaming jet by his daily dollop of Brylcreem. Its blackness is a betrayal of a family secret that somewhere in a distant branch of his family tree there lurked, like a monkey poised to disrupt family mythology, a liaison between a European man and an Indian woman. His dark brown eyes are concealed behind thick rectangular glasses; his lips are unusually full and sensuous for a man. The only signs of his age are a few streaks of silver in his hair and a slight paunch drooping over his belt. He carries a fold-up aluminium garden chair towards a circular concrete patio in the shade of the house.

As he moves, I notice a slight stoop in his normally erect bearing, a reminder of his youthful athletic days. As he bends to unfold the chair, he winces. He lowers himself slowly, then shifts and squirms. He can't seem to find a comfortable position. Thinking himself unobserved, his face contorts into a grimace. Beads of sweat sprout on his forehead.

My inner doctor awakes: this man's in serious pain.

My mother, a short, plump woman in her late sixties, pads into the kitchen. She's wearing a frilly nightcap, fluffy housecoat, and slippers, which make her look like a nursemaid straight from Dickens. Like my father, she has bad eyesight, and wears tear-drop shaped frames which magnify her tiny cornflower-blue eyes.

"Good morning. Coffee, darling?"

As she plugs in the kettle, she notices my stare.

"Oh yes. He's been in terrible pain for the past month. I've been trying to get him to go see someone about it, but he won't go."

My father's just like other doctors I've met. So quick to diagnose their patients, so stubborn about getting their own symptoms looked at. Do physicians really think they have enough objectivity to make self-diagnoses? Do they fear appearing weak and vulnerable to colleagues? Or are they afraid of turning into the dreaded "other" – a patient? For a doctor, becoming a patient can be terrifying because this patient can't be shielded from the truth.

"Why don't you speak to him? Perhaps he'll listen to another doctor."

I nod, but the idea of confronting my father panics me. It's not that he's tyrannical or autocratic – far from it. He is often quiet to the point of being a shadow. He's an intensely private person who rebuffs any attempt to find out how he's feeling or what he's thinking. Any enquiry into his wellness will encounter a polite but firm barrier first erected during a sometimes harsh boyhood in the boarding schools of colonial India.

She scoops instant coffee crystals into three mugs, and splashes hot water over them. The aroma of coffee fills the kitchen.

"It's a lovely warm day," she says. "Why don't we join Daddy outside?"

We carry the mugs and a plate of biscuits to the patio. I unfold two additional chairs, and we sit. The warmth of the autumnal sun is delicious. Trixie weaves nervously around the lawn, sniffing the grass.

"Your garden's looking good," I say.

"Thank you," my father smiles.

"After he retires, he'll have more time to spend out here," my mother says, nibbling on her biscuit.

Trixie crouches and delivers a shiny chocolate-brown turd onto the lawn. My father emits a "tut-tut" and, placing both hands on the armrests to push himself up, starts to rise from his chair.

I stand up. "I'll get it."

"No," he says with a firmness that makes both Trixie and me sit.

He shuffles to the tool shed and grabs a spade. He scrapes the beagle's gift off the lawn and tosses it into the flower bed, where it lands at the feet of the Edwardian ladies. They shudder.

As he returns to us, something about the severity of his limp strikes a chord of familiarity. Yes, it's just like one of my cancer patients hobbling around the examining room. For the first time I think, My God, maybe my father's got cancer.

"Are you okay?" I say.

"Fine," he mutters.

"No, you're not." Crumbs tumble from my mother's lips. "Tell Charles about your pain."

"I don't have pain."

"He's been living on Tylenols."

He carefully lowers himself back into the chair and gives a dismissive flick of the hand.

"It's just arthritis."

Over the brim of her cup, my mother's eyes focus on me in a pleading stare. Trixie nuzzles against my shin, and I drop my gaze to meet her brown, inquisitive eyes. I dare not speak my mind. After all, what do I know? My father's a rehabilitation doctor, an expert in bones, joints, and muscles. My oncology lens is warped. In my business, *everyone* with pain has cancer. Not all pain is cancer, I remind myself.

There's another factor operating in my reticence. Despite the array of diplomas on my office wall, in the presence of my father I still don't feel like a Real Doctor.

At birth, medicine seemed to be my destiny. My paternal grandfather, Robert, was born in India and trained in medicine at Grant Medical College, Bombay. He served as an army medic in the dirty campaigns of France and the Middle East during World War I. Later, he was awarded the MBE – Member of the Most Excellent Order of the British Empire – for his administration of the Calcutta School of Tropical Medicine during the interwar years. His wife, Kathleen, my future grandmother, was the daughter of another colonial Indian doctor. After World War II and Indian independence, my grandparents settled in England – where my father had already been sent to boarding school. For them, England was a drab, chilly foreign country far removed from the warmth and colour of India.

My mother, Joyce, was of sturdy, Protestant, God-fearing, middle-class southern English stock. After helping her teenaged brother (and my future favourite uncle) Edgar recover from measles encephalitis, she was encouraged to enter nursing. Russell, quiet and studious, and Joyce, boisterous and outspoken, collided in the operating rooms at Bart's Hospital, London, when she was a student nurse and he a junior doctor. They married in 1950.

In my childhood home, there were reminders of Medicine – or "Med'Sin," as my mother pronounced it, hissing the sibilant at anyone who dared challenge its supreme position in the professional universe. A massive dog-eared copy of *Grey's Anatomy*, with neat marginalia and underlinings in blue-black ink from my father's fountain pen, rested on the bookshelf, next to a textbook of forensic medicine with gruesome photographs of electrocuted, burned, or slashed dead people. For as long as I can remember, a battered wooden box lay under my parents' bed. It contained a collection of human bones, a souvenir of my father's anatomy studies. Occasionally, my father allowed my sister and me to handle them. I remember the wispy strings of dried sinew fluttering off the humerus like the flayed catgut of a broken bowstring. There was also a skull with yellow teeth rattling in the jaw. The cranium flipped open to reveal the empty chamber that once held a brain. These objects were playthings: never once did we discuss that they might once have been part of a living, breathing, dreaming human being. I learned early on a skill vital in medicine: detachment from horror.

If I felt the powerful pull of family gravity towards "Med'Sin," I also felt a tug from a more distant universe. Somewhere out there, there was a star: James Hayter, a portly, fruity-voiced character actor of the mid-twentieth century, who built his film reputation on portraying rotund jovial characters such as Mr. Pickwick and Friar Tuck. He can be glimpsed as the bookseller in the film version of *Oliver!* I've never been able to establish with certainty that we're related, but his birth in India and physical resemblance to family members makes it very likely.

I shared his theatrical genes. My earliest ambition was to become a circus clown. As a boy, I acquired a collection of marionettes and put on shows for my long-suffering family and friends; in high school, I acted in plays and became president of the Drama Club. I didn't dislike science; I devoured every issue of *Science Digest* and shared in the general wonder at the discoveries of the late twentieth century and the bright future they offered, but I found something about science's rootedness in fact and measurement to be mind-numbingly plodding and prosaic. I preferred the unconstrained, rich life of the imagination, which had been awoken by reading Carroll and Dickens and stimulated by some excellent teachers. When I headed off to university at Queen's University, Kingston, it was to study English and drama with the intent, perhaps, of eventually becoming an actor. In a curious foreshadowing of my life, Theological Hall at Queen's housed both the Drama Department and the Medical Library. As I read, discussed, and rehearsed plays, I glimpsed the earnest, textbook-laden medical students scurrying up and down the circular library stairs.

Something held me back from full commitment to a theatrical career. Always a bit shy and reserved, I lacked the unashamedly large egos and bumptious self-confidence of many of my drama classmates. With the clarity of hindsight, I see I was wrestling with homosexual feelings and was worried the intimacy of interactions in the theatre would force me to reveal more of myself than I dared. I decided to enter the more cloistered life of a theatre academic, so I headed west to the University of Calgary, where, after writing a thesis on Victorian comedy, I obtained an MA in drama. I then landed back at Queen's University as an instructor in drama. As the newbie, I was assigned to teach the department's first-ever course in Canadian theatre. I spent one glorious summer teaching drama at Bermuda College, where I was thrilled to awaken a genuine interest in theatre in students such as police officers who perceived drama as an easy elective. It marked the beginning of my lifelong love of teaching.

Already I could feel my trajectory losing momentum. I wasn't sure I wanted the sedentary, introspective life of an academic. By now I was married to a vivacious and creative woman who'd been an undergraduate classmate, and we had one child. These realities forced a major rethink of my path. What next? For a while I felt weightless, spinning, tumbling through space, with no obvious direction.

In *When Breath Becomes Air*, neurosurgeon Dr. Paul Kalanithi describes how his craving for direct experience of life after years of studying literature propelled him to medicine. For me, the life event that pivoted me homewards to medicine was the birth of my daughter, Rosalind, in 1978. Sitting in the delivery room, squeezing my wife's hand, observing the primal, painful, yet joyous process, I witnessed something more wondrous, miraculous, and real compared to anything I'd experienced in the theatre. Other than a painful skirmish with an anal fissure as a graduate student, it was the first moment in my life when I'd witnessed the practice of medicine up close, from the bedside of a patient. As I watched the doctors and nurses ministering to my wife over many hours of difficult labour, I felt a tug, a pull, a calling – one so strong it seemed as though doctoring had merely laid dormant in my bones like cancer cells in remission.

The tug also came from a different direction: a need to connect with my father. Like Kalanithi, son of a cardiologist, in my early life "I knew medicine only by its absence." First in England, later in Canada, my father was preoccupied with his medical career. Even when present at home, he was often detached, sitting apart, lost in thought, quietly taking deep draughts from a cigarette, blue smoke wreathing his anxious forehead. I had glimpses of the kind, gentle soul beneath, but some mysterious internal oppression held him back from spontaneity or joy.

My mother's frustration at his passivity and withdrawal sometimes erupted in tantrums. But for the most part, nobody complained. This is how it is to be the children of a doctor. Everyone in the family has to put their needs second. You just have to suck it up. Remember that Daddy is pursuing the highest calling of all, one that involves sacrifice for everyone. Leave him alone, don't bother him, he's tired from work and needs to rest. Yet I still felt a deep-seated yearning for connection, and thought medicine might create that bond.

It turned out to be an opportune time for a drama graduate to seek entry to medical school. In the late 1970s, medical schools were rethinking their admissions criteria. Since the early twentieth century, medical training had been firmly rooted in sciences such as biochemistry and physiology. At the time I did my undergraduate drama degree, medical schools accepted students, as they did in my father's day, directly from high school into a two-year "pre-med" program heavily weighted to science. This program led immediately to four years of med school and the MD degree.

In the 1970s, this educational path was starting to be seen as insufficient. While it produced physicians skilled at diagnosis and intervention, it did not always result in doctors capable of dealing with the complex emotional and social needs of their patients. Science also coated doctors with a varnish of hubris that led to a public perception of doctors as cold and arrogant, a perception that came into crisp focus during the later fights for abortion rights and AIDS treatments. The public wanted doctors who were well-rounded individuals who could be sensitive to their patients as human beings, not just cases of disease. As a result, many schools rethought their admissions criteria and by the time I applied had changed their basic entry requirement to full completion of an undergraduate degree in any subject, as long as the basic science courses had been completed along the way. (Some schools, such as McMaster in Hamilton, Ontario, went further and jettisoned the science requirement completely.) Although these changes extended the period to graduation with an MD from six to eight years, they were supposed to result in more compassionate, well-rounded doctors.

So when I nervously entered the admission dean's office for a preliminary chat about the possibility of a drama graduate entering medical school, I was surprised and pleased at his warm and encouraging response. I floundered on the science-based MCAT, but my undergraduate and graduate academic standing was enough to gain offers of acceptance at several medical schools. Within a year, I became one of those earnest, textbook-toting medical students I'd glimpsed at Queen's University.

Because I hadn't taken any science courses during my previous undergraduate degree, I had to take crash basic courses in biology, physics, chemistry, and organic chemistry before I could begin. So I fired up my retro-rockets and made a bumpy, rattling descent from the stratosphere of the arts to first-year science courses. The journey was softer than expected. After years of education in the humanities, with reams of readings, essay writings, and seminar discussions, I found the old-fashioned rote learning style of the basic sciences, and then in the early years of medical school, rather dull and unchallenging. It was the sheer volume of new information that was daunting. My acting background came in handy, for it had given me skills at memorization.

The descent became bumpier when I arrived in the wards of the hospital for the first time. Like all medical students in the transition between book and bedside teaching, I suddenly confronted the limitations of the facts I'd so assiduously memorized. I was faced with patients who had unexplainable symptoms, unrelieved suffering, or were even dying. It was often hard to fit patients into the neat diagnostic categories outlined in my lecture notes.

Beyond this, my inner humanist, cultivated through my education in the arts, revolted at the sight of how the medical system ground human beings down to faceless "cases." I saw why the public was clamouring for a change in medical attitudes and a new set of admissions criteria. The reductionism of modern medicine is a well-worn trope but it is a trope rooted firmly in truth. With few exceptions, my clinician-professors regarded patients as mere specimens of diseases and had little interest in them as human beings. The hospital was a great assembly line of healing, its labs and diagnostic facilities reducing patients to diagnoses that had somehow to be "managed." I survived this inhumane atmosphere like most medical students: by conforming, adopting the language and comportment of my teachers, and assuming the role of Doctor. But beneath my white coat I continued to feel disheartened and occasionally disgusted at the inhumanity of the medical machine.

I was determined to enter a field of medicine where I could put my previous education in the humanities to good use, and maybe, at least in my own practice, even redress some of the inhumanity I'd seen. Psychiatry seemed the obvious choice, but I became quickly disappointed after some elective stints. It was an era when the third edition of the *Diagnostic and Statistical Manual of Mental Disorders* (DSM-III) reigned supreme, and most of the psychiatrists I met were more interested in thumbing through this biblical tome to fix the patient in the crosshairs of a neat diagnostic axis than actually listening to the nuances of their life stories. The emphasis on classification, categorization, biochemical explanations, and pill pushing turned me off.

At first glance, radiation oncology was not an obvious choice for a former drama instructor intent on satisfying his latent humanities instincts. In the summer between the second and third years of medical school, I did a placement at the Kingston, Ontario, Regional Cancer Centre, and there had my first taste of the field. Up to that point, I had, like most medical students, a dim conception of radiotherapy. What's that? Something given to dying cancer patients to ease their passage into death? Involving huge machines that gyrate, whir, and discharge painful "zaps"? By geeky doctors more interested in calculating beam angles than caring for patients? The environment proved more cheerful and humane than I expected. Instead of dying, many patients were cured of cancer using radiation alone. Others were elated when symptoms from cancer abated after radiation. Those big, scary machines turned out to be creative instruments of hope for sick humans.

Above all, I encountered doctors whose compassion, patience, and humour set them as far apart from the geeky stereotype as possible. I remember vividly my surprise – and immediate unease – at spotting one of the male radiation oncologists, Dr. Friar, a tall, burly, Falstaffian figure who later became one of my mentors, sitting at the bedside of a patient with metastatic breast cancer, discussing her situation while simultaneously gently stroking her hand. My unease, the product of many months of witnessing the distant, often brusque behaviour of my teachers – doctors aren't supposed to stroke patients' hands! – quickly melted into admiration for his openness and kindness. It was astonishing that radiation oncologists like him could be more empathic than the psychiatrists I met. Their work took place in an environment of complicated technology, but they were, first and foremost, sensitive, caring clinicians for whom radiotherapy was a tool, not an end in itself. During that summer, I also spent a couple of weeks with the social service nurses – the forerunners of today's palliative care nurses. With them, I got an up-close look at the complex emotional dramas following in the wake of a cancer diagnosis.

It seemed that radiation oncology might satisfy my inner yearnings to fuse my arts background with my medical training. I toyed with entering another specialty such as internal medicine, but, with its endless number-crunching of laboratory data, it seemed too abstract. Besides, internists, while wizards at making clever diagnoses, had few genuine treatments up their sleeves. A lot of internal medicine seemed to boil down to prescribing prednisone, a steroid, to cut inflammation. I had witnessed radiation's ability to actually cure patients. I might have chosen family medicine, but it seemed dull compared to the high-stakes arena of the cancer centre.

Radiation oncology fit in another way. By the time I graduated from medical school, I was the father of two young children. I was determined not to reenact my father's absence from my childhood life. In the late 1980s, post-graduate training in radiation oncology could be completed in three years after internship, and the bulk of the clinical work occurred in regular working hours. Unlike other specialties, I didn't have to stay in the hospital on evenings or weekends when I was on call. This arrangement would allow me to spend time with my family, and I hoped I could give my children the attention that had been missing from my own childhood.

Like my father's field of rehabilitation medicine, radiation oncology was not a glamorous specialty and did not attract many candidates. My interest was welcomed enthusiastically, and I was accepted immediately into the training program.

Over three years, I learned the unique body of knowledge of radiation oncology. Most practising radiation oncologists specialize in only three or four types of cancer, but as a trainee I had to master the geography, taxonomy, and behaviour of every type of malignant infestation of the human body: their species, subspecies, and "natural history" – the process through which, undetected and unchecked, they spread, choking out healthy tissues and organs and ultimately invading other territories. Each cancer has its own favourite pattern of spread, such as the predilection of prostate cancer to colonize bones without appearing anywhere else, or melanoma of the eye, which can unexpectedly show up in the liver. I had to learn these nuances of spread for both common and rare cancers, and how to assign a "stage" to a patient's cancer. "Staging" is the process of determining the extent of cancer in the body from the results of physical examination, imaging studies, and lab tests. Because every cancer has a unique pattern of spread, each has its own stage classification system. Little did this former drama teacher anticipate that within a few years, he'd find himself immersed in a different kind of staging.

I also had to master concepts of radiation physics and radiobiology essential to understanding the application of radiation to humans. In retrospect, it seems almost a miracle an arts graduate grasped concepts such as the Compton Effect and Relative Biological Effectiveness. I survived because of the excellence and patience of my teachers, and also because I saw radiotherapy was, to a large extent, art that involved much creativity – such as the "Elastoplast mould" devised by one of my mentors to treat an ugly, recalcitrant skin cancer on the back of a patient's hand. It was basically a sticky bandage impregnated with radioactive pellets strapped to the hand for a few hours. Its apparent simplicity belied careful calculations preventing over-irradiation of the delicate underlying tissues. A few months later, the cancer was gone and – presto! – the skin healed to pink baby-like smoothness. Such apparent miracles encouraged my learning of the background science.

With the support of excellent clinical teachers, I passed my examinations in radiation oncology in 1988. I began my career at the Saint John Regional Hospital, a brand-new facility on a promontory overlooking the Saint John River in New Brunswick. It was a great place to start. Later, like most radiation oncologists, I would become a subspecialist in only three or four types of cancer, but in Saint John I was a GP-radiation oncologist and saw whatever cases were assigned to me. One week, I saw cases of larynx, bladder, and breast cancer, the next, lung, thyroid, or brain cancer. I also had a smattering of patients with rare tumours I'd only read about in textbooks, such as the chordoma, a slow-growing tumour of the spine, an oncological oddity, the bane of radiation oncology trainees because of its frequent appearance in examination questions.

It was both exhilarating and terrifying to finally be in charge of patients' care. During my training, a senior staff member had always supervised my decisions. Now, here I was, a newly graduated Rad Onc, wobbling alone on the pivot of a see-saw between cure and toxicity. I saw a young French-Canadian man with an advanced, inoperable tumour slowly eating its way through his nasal passages and sinuses. I could cure him with radiation, but I was terrified I might destroy his eyes or liquefy part of his brain.

So, on that sunny September morning in Calgary, when I sit with my parents in their garden, silently wondering about my father's pain – as I am certain they are too – I have much to be proud of: I've graduated from medical school and from a specialist training program, and I have several months of independent practice under my belt. Already I've supported many patients and their families through the ordeal of radiation treatment. I couldn't have done all this without the unflagging support of my wife and the joy of my two children.

And yet, somehow, I still don't feel like a Real Doctor. As I stare at my father, wanting to ask him more about his pain following the algorithm of questions I ask my own patients, and to encourage him to get some tests done, a profound sense of inadequacy bubbles up. How can I, a drama dilettante turned doctor, challenge a man who has a real mastery of science and decades more experience than me? As my mother loves to declare, my father is a "Senior Doctor." I'm at best his junior, a neophyte, a rookie.

The next day, I fly home to New Brunswick. The question of the cause of my father's pain remains unresolved.

2

The Reticent Doctor

Cancer is an unruly and demanding intruder. If its complaints are neglected, it shrieks more loudly and shrilly until its host has no choice but to turn and recognize its presence.

Over the fall, my father's pain becomes so severe he finally agrees to see a doctor and have some tests.

Christmas 1989: He and my mother make the long trek from Calgary to Saint John for a holiday visit. My mother bears an envelope with his results in her purse.

At the airport, I notice his careful, measured step and firm grip on the rail as he descends from the jet to the snowy tarmac. He's only just turned sixty-five, but he suddenly looks like a frail old man. Uncharacteristically, he allows me to carry his bag to the car.

Later that evening, after we've eaten a Christmas Eve supper of ham and mince tarts, and my wife has taken our two children upstairs to bed, my parents and I sit in the living room, our shins warmed by the heat of a blazing fire, sipping glasses of sherry and nibbling on shortbread. Our black mutt Tessie lies in a doggy coma by the hearth. A program of Christmas carols wafts from the radio. Outside, the snow swirls and settles into smooth white drifts as high as the sills.

My mother sets her glass aside, heaves herself from her comfy chair, and disappears for a few minutes. When she returns, she's carrying the bulging envelope bearing the tidings.

"Not now," growls my father.

"I want this over with," she says, thrusting the envelope at me.

I pull a sheaf of papers out. My eyes immediately rest on the conclusion of an X-ray report: "*an osteoblastic focus in the lumbar vertebrae.*"

Osteo-blastic: from the Greek *ostos*, bone, and *blastos*, germ. A germ in the bone.

It's a term I know well.

"Tell me what this shows," my examiner, a tall, elegantly dressed man with an upright bearing not unlike my father's, said a little more than a year earlier during my oral examination in radiation oncology, as he pinned an X-ray of an unknown patient's spine to a view box.

I immediately recognized the white ice balls cascading through the patient's spine.

"*Osteoblastic foci* in the bones," I said in my careful, well-rehearsed manner.

His lips pressed in a thin smile.

Osteoblasts. Bone germs. Malignant germs.

Malignant germs so dense, so greedy, they absorb all the energy from the X-rays, preventing darkening of the radiation-sensitive silver film beneath, leaving empty white spheres on the plate. Sometimes the whiteness fills the bone so completely they become *ivory vertebrae.*

Ivory, like the dainty carved trinkets from India adorning my grandmother's apartment.

My father now has his own ivory treasures. A white colonizer of his bones.

My hunch in the garden was right. My father has cancer in his spine. No wonder his pain was so bad.

I daren't look up and meet my parents' gaze just yet. I shuffle through the other reports and find a lab test showing a raised level of acid phosphatase, an enzyme secreted by the prostate, in the blood.

The twin findings of ivory vertebrae and raised acid phosphatase are enough to clinch a diagnosis of metastatic prostate cancer. Germs from a cancerous prostate have infected my father's spine.

I'm aware of my parents' eyes fixed on me, waiting for my response. These worried, searching looks are familiar from encounters in the consulting rooms of the cancer clinic, as patients, their partners, and children look to me for answers about a situation.

How much do they know? What has his doctor in Calgary told him? Has he pussy-footed around the truth? Has he brushed them off with one of those vague statements such as "There're a few shadows on the bone"?

But no. My father's a doctor, my mother's a nurse, both with their own X-ray vision capable of seeing through obfuscation. Besides, they must have looked at these reports themselves. They know. In that case, what do they expect me to say? Are they looking to me for a second opinion? For reassurance? A glimmer of hope? Or merely for someone to share the burden with?

Paralysis settles over my body, as if I've just been injected with a sedative. It's a strangely familiar feeling, connected to that detachment I felt handling the bones under my parents' bed and the blithe chatter about medical conditions I've heard from my parents at the dinner table.

A surge of "God Rest Ye Merry Gentlemen" loosens the paralysis. I take a deep breath and look up at my parents' faces. Through the flickering reflections of the fire on their glasses I glimpse my mother's eyes narrowed in anxiety, my father's alight with curiosity.

The carol comes to an end. There's no sound but the crackle of logs in the fire and the moan of the wind outside.

No one in this triad of Senior Doctor, Junior Doctor, and Nurse dares to speak the name of the invader aloud.

In the final year of medical school, my classmates and I leap the gulf between theoretical and practical learning to become clinical clerks, senior medical students who assist in the care of hospital inpatients. Our short white jackets and wide-eyed enthusiasm distinguish us from the weary and often cynical long-coated residents who supervise us. At the time I went to medical school, the clinical clerk was the lowliest serf of the medical hierarchy and was expected, with little direct training and almost no supervision, to perform tedious, repetitive, and sometimes repugnant tasks – "scut work" – such as writing up admission histories, chasing up lab results, and inserting needles or tubes into bodily orifices. It was all based on antiquated ideas, redolent of military academies or Victorian boarding schools, of building "character" and learning by osmosis rather than structured education. From what I glean from talking to current medical students, little has changed over the years.

Early in my clerkship year I spend two months on a surgical ward. The surgical rotation is the most demanding of all, with visits to drowsy patients at the crack of dawn followed by endless hours in the operating room holding retractors at uncomfortable angles as a short-tempered surgeon excavates a body cavity. In the operating room, the clerk, referred to as "the slug," often receives sharp prods if there's even a slight drift of the retractor. At the end of the day, the clerk goes back to the ward to write up admission histories on newly admitted patients. The work frequently extends into the evening hours.

Like today: It's 7:00 p.m., and, hoping to exit so I can enjoy a bike ride home by the lake, I'm in the cramped office behind the nursing station, tucking my clerk jacket into my knapsack. A nurse whose face is a mask of fatigue appears at the door and slumps against the frame.

"Don't go yet, hon. There's a new admission needs a history and physical."

"Oh. Isn't there anyone else to do it?"

"'Fraid not, hon. Everyone else is tied up with an emergency case in the OR."

She hands me a clipboard with the admission forms and wanders away. I understand her predicament: she can't start her nursing care for the patient until there's a history and preliminary orders written in the chart. I open my knapsack, unfold my jacket, and glance through the paperwork.

Fifty-four-year-old man. Admitting diagnosis: stomach cancer.

I stick a notepad and pen into my pocket, sling my stethoscope around my neck, and march to the patient's room. My heart thuds, and a sticky film forms between my palm and the clipboard. Stomach cancer? My book learning taught me it's a particularly unpleasant malignancy that produces nasty symptoms such as vomiting blood. It's usually detected at an advanced stage and is rarely cured. I expect to encounter an obviously ill, even emaciated person. But at only fifty-four? I'm not sure how to react or what to say.

Have I gone to the wrong room? Sam is a youthful looking man with a broad face anchored by prominent cheekbones and surmounted by a tussle of black hair. He's sitting cross-legged on his bed, leafing through a magazine. His legs, poking sideways from his flimsy blue hospital gown, are beefy as a soccer player's. I recognize the letters in the magazine as Korean.

He looks up at me, gives me a warm smile, and lays the magazine aside. "Hi!"

From somewhere in my memory I recall a Korean greeting a friend taught me.

"Ann-yong-ha-say-o!"

He grins. "You know Korean?"

I shrug. "That's about it."

He laughs. "Good start, though."

"I'm the medical student. I'm here to do your history and physical."

"Have a seat," he says, indicating the chair.

I sit, flip open my notebook, and begin to take his history. His friendliness makes my job easier. He tells me he's an airline pilot, the son of immigrants who came to Canada after the Korean War. He lives with his partner, Sylvia, and has two children from a first marriage. A few weeks ago during an overseas flight, he developed this "bad belly ache – right here," he says, jabbing his fingers in the inverted-V shaped space between the lower ribs.

Thinking it might be recurrence of stomach ulcers of a few years earlier, his family doctor had started him on acid reducers, but the pain had not gone away. About a week ago, Sam developed constant nausea, which left him unable to ingest anything other than sports drinks and liquid supplements. His doctor ordered a barium swallow, a type of X-ray involving drinking dye to outline the stomach. The test showed "something in the stomach," so he was referred to a gastroenterologist, who performed a scope and took biopsies.

I know from the pathology report clipped to his notes that the biopsies showed a typical form of stomach cancer, adenocarcinoma – from the Greek *adeno*, gland, because the cells resemble the glands secreting stomach juices.

Sam sighs. "It looks like the ulcers are back. This time I need them removed."

My gaze drops to the clipboard. He doesn't know he has cancer?

"Uh, is that what the GI doctor said?" I ask.

"He didn't say anything. His secretary called to say I needed to see a surgeon."

Without any warning, Sam's abdomen heaves. His eyes widen, and he points to a kidney basin on the window sill. I grab it, place it under his chin, and he spews slimy red liquid into it. The room fills with the acrid stench of stagnant stomach fluids.

"Hold on," I say, "let me get some help."

I trot to the nursing station and consult with my senior, the resident, Jeff, a sandy-haired man whose freckled baby face hides an often snarky demeanour. He's just returned from the OR. His normally pink face is grey, and his greens are stained and rumpled, like he's just survived a battle.

"Put in an N-G tube?" he says, with a shrug and a questioning tone, like I should have known better than ask him what to do.

An N-G (nasogastric tube) is a plastic tube threaded through the nose down into the stomach and attached to a suction machine. Its purpose is to relieve pressure when the stomach is not emptying properly. I go to the utility room, search in the jumble of baskets for the tubing and pump, and carry it back to Sam's room.

There's a motto that describes clerkship training for medical procedures: "Watch one, do one, teach one" – meaning all that is necessary before performing a procedure is to watch someone else do it, then have someone else watch you as you do it. I had inserted a couple of N-G tubes on my own, not always with great success. Just after I inserted the tube into the nose of an elderly woman, her face morphed into a gorgon-like mask and her teeth protruded through her lips. Coiled round her palate, the tube was pushing her dentures out. On my next case, I adopted the tone of a flight attendant ordering passengers to brace and commanded the patient to "swallow! swallow! swallow!" as soon as he felt the tickle of the end of the tube in his throat. The tube slid in easily.

Sam's tube slides in with similar ease. I attach it to the suction machine and flip the on switch. There's a gurgling and swishing as the suction pulls the frothy, blood-specked liquid to a jar. Sam flops back on his pillow and gives me a weak smile.

"Thanks. That feels better."

I leave him to rest. I retreat to the back office and write up my notes in his chart. Dodging Jeff, who might come up with more work for me to do, I quickly pack my knapsack and escape.

As I cycle home through the gathering dusk, weaving through the late spring air infused with the scent of lilacs, I think of Sam's situation. How could someone so apparently fit have cancer? Maybe the diagnosis is wrong. But no, the name on the report was correct and the diagnosis was very clear. To be sure, that violent retching points to something much more sinister than ulcers.

If he does have cancer, why doesn't he know? He seems to think he has ulcers that can be removed with surgery. I can't believe the gastroenterologist didn't inform him in person of the results. Maybe he did, and Sam's in denial. But there was no hint of evasion in response to my questions.

What if he really doesn't know the truth? If so, who's going to tell him? It can't be up to me, the lowliest member of the team. Surely such important information should be delivered by Dr. McCutcheon, the surgeon in charge of his case. How will he deliver the news? How will Sam take it? Even from our brief encounter, I can see he's a nice fellow, and I don't want him hurt. I imagine my own shock at learning of my own body's betrayal. Can he be told in a way that's gentle and respectful? In second year of medical school, we'd had brief pointers on "breaking bad news," but they seem inadequate in the face of the devastating nature of Sam's diagnosis.

I'm back on the ward at 6:30 a.m. Promptly at 6:45 a.m., Dr. McCutcheon emerges through the swing doors at the end of the ward. He's a tall, bald man of about sixty, with a military bearing and a scowl permanently etched on his face. Though the nurses don't stand to attention as they did in my mother's day, I notice they stiffen at his appearance.

Jeff, I, and the nurse in charge form a line in front of the desk.

"Any new patients?" he snaps.

"Yes, sir." I begin to review Sam's history, starting with his family background. "Stomach cancer is more prevalent in the Asian population," I announce, beaming as I proudly show off this new piece of information I'd gleaned from a textbook the night before.

McCutcheon closes his eyes and sighs. "Don't waste my time." He turns to Jeff. "Let's see the films."

Jeff leads us to the back room, where he pins Sam's X-rays to a view box. He points out the glistening white snake of barium dye uncoiling from the throat, sliding through the oesophagus, and finally collapsed in a heap in the stomach, where it ends in a tangled, chaotic coil, like the snake consuming itself. I've seen X-ray images of stomach cancer in textbooks, but this is the first time I'm face to face with it in a real live person. In the context of knowing the pleasant man to whom these images belong, its twisted form seems especially malevolent.

McCutcheon rips the X-rays from the view box, shoves them into an envelope, and turns to me.

"What's the plan, son?"

"Uh, operate?" I stutter.

Jeff snorts. "Duh? No kidding. Welcome to surgery, doctor."

The three of us troop to Sam's room. He's lying in bed, gazing at a TV screen suspended from a frame.

Seeing us, he turns off the TV, sits up, and smiles warmly.

"Morning, docs," he says brightly.

"Morning," says Jeff. "This is Dr. McCutcheon, your surgeon."

Dr. McCutcheon emits a grunt of greeting, leans over, lifts the bed-sheets, and pokes Sam's belly. Sam winces.

Dr. McCutcheon straightens and says, "We'll book you for the OR tomorrow."

"Sure, doc. I want this over and done with."

McCutcheon pivots towards the door. Jeff follows.

"Oh, doc. It is just ulcers, isn't it?"

McCutcheon and Jeff freeze. After a moment, their heads swivel back.

I hold my breath. We've arrived at the moment of truth. Lying alone in the bed, Sam suddenly seems small and vulnerable. I contain an urge to sit on the bed beside him.

Dr. McCutcheon's scowl morphs into a Punch-like mask of fake cheeriness.

"It's just a growth," he says, waving his hand. His light-hearted tone is that of a landscaper describing an unwelcome weed at the end of a garden.

Sam's brows knit. "You'll get rid of it?" he says.

The fibres of Dr. McCutcheon's cheek twitch, betraying a clenching of the jaw.

"See you tomorrow," says Jeff.

I follow the surgeons from the room. As we leave I glance back at Sam. He's lying back on his pillow, gazing at the ceiling, brows knitted more tightly.

I trot down the corridor behind Jeff and McCutcheon. Why hasn't the surgeon told Sam directly he has cancer? The vague word "growth" did not begin to capture the ominous nature of Sam's illness.

"Er ... he speaks perfect English, you know," I blurt.

The two surgeons either don't hear me or pretend not to hear. Without replying, they turn quickly into the next patient's room.

Later that afternoon, after a five-hour stint in the OR where I've been peppered with questions about the gallbladder over the anesthetized belly of a woman undergoing its removal, I visit Sam again. His partner, Sylvia, is there. She's a tiny, thin woman, perhaps in her midforties. Her navy suit, scarf of red and blue stripes, and wing-shaped badge give away her occupation as flight attendant.

As soon as I enter, she stands up. "Finally. I came here straight off a red-eye. I've been waiting since then to talk to someone."

She fixes me with dark brown eyes. "Sam says he's got a growth in his stomach? What exactly does that mean?"

I teeter lightly on my heels. "Ummm ... well, you'll have to discuss that with Dr. McCutcheon. He's in charge."

"The nurse says he can't be reached. Why can't you tell me? What exactly does Sam have?"

Their intensely curious gazes pin me to the wall.

"Well, it does look like a growth of some kind."

"Does that mean it's cancer?"

The walls of my throat flutter.

"I, uh ... uh ..."

Sam tugs at Sylvia's sleeve.

"Leave him alone, Sylvia. He's just a student."

"He must know."

I'm saved by a nurse entering to adjust Sam's IV.

"I've got to run," I blurt. "I'll see if the resident is around. He's better at explaining than me."

Jeff is nowhere to be found. As I sit in the back room, riffling through a pile of lab reports, my cheeks burn with shame. Sam and Sylvia deserve the truth. I could have told them. Why didn't I? Was I afraid? Afraid of messing it up, of upsetting them, of making them angry? Maybe even afraid of reprisal for overstepping my bounds as a lowly student?

Sam's situation was the first of many occasions when I observed the curtain of silence doctors drop around the word cancer.

After I completed my Canadian training in radiation, I worked for six months at the Royal Marsden Hospital in London, England. The Marsden is a famous hospital where many cancer luminaries work, including one who was a world-renowned expert in cancers of the throat and mouth. I was thrilled to work with a doctor whose important papers I'd read during my earlier training.

He turned out to be the very model of a tweedy British professor, a corona of wispy hairs around a bald head, smudged spectacles dangling on his nose, a pipe bowl poking like a periscope from the breast pocket of a worn, rumpled jacket.

One afternoon, I stood behind him and gazed over his shoulder as he used a pair of wooden tongue depressors to pry open the mouth of an unkempt, unshaven man reeking of stale tobacco. As the professor swivelled his own head to focus the beam from his headlamp into the throat, the light picked out the bloated, ragged crimson face of a large cancer in the right tonsil. The beast stared back, as if angry at being disturbed from its slumber in the cave. Using the end of the tongue depressor, the professor poked the cancer and released rivulets of pus that dripped onto the patient's tongue. I teetered back as nauseating fumes of rotting meat reached my nose. A swelling like mumps on the exterior of the patient's neck told me the cancer had taken deep root in the surrounding tissues and lymph nodes.

As if performing a vocal warm-up, the professor emitted a sing-song-like "Uuuh-huum," withdrew his tongue depressors, switched off his headlamp, and said with a plummy, cheery English accent, "Well, you've got a spot of trouble there."

I could hardly believe my ears. A spot of "trouble"? The poor man had very advanced cancer. I knew even the most heroic surgery and radiation offered a slim chance of cure.

"We'll fix up that trouble in no time," he said, with a pat on the patient's knee. He stood up, stripped off his headlamp, and made a swift exit, leaving the patient to gaze after him with an open mouth of puzzlement.

Through my whole month tagging along with him, the professor never once used the word "cancer." It was always "trouble."

McCutcheon's "growth" and the professor's "trouble" are just two of many examples from an entire sub-vocabulary of oncologic obfuscation:

"There's a *swelling* in your groin."
"There appears to be a *shadow* in your lung."
"There are some *spots* in the liver."
"It looks like there's a *mass* in the colon."
"I saw a *lesion* in the bladder."
"It appears we are dealing with a *neoplastic process*."
"The *bad cells* are taking over."

Why is cancer such a loaded word, a chunk of gristle that gets trapped in the gorge of doctors and replaced by sweet mushy candy-words? To answer this question it's helpful to look at medical history. Up until the early twentieth century, cancer was an insignificant blip on the radar of medicine. Diseases such as cholera, syphilis, and tuberculosis, once thought to originate from vague environmental "miasmas," preoccupied doctors. The advent of the germ theory of disease and the discovery of specific causative bacteria helped to usher in a new scientific, laboratory-based approach that led to the development of rational, targeted therapies such as antibiotics. As treatments for tuberculosis and syphilis improved, their significance declined, and other diseases, such as cancer, moved to the forefront of public and medical attention. But, as suggested by the title of American historian James Patterson's study of cancer and American culture, *The Dread Disease*, cancer arrived with significant emotional baggage. First, it was a mysterious process, the body's unpredictable and frightening revolt against itself: as one commentator said, cancer cells were the rogue "Bolshevik cells" of the body. Second, despite advances in surgery and radiotherapy, no treatment was seen as effective, so the disease resulted in an unrelenting downward course of unremitting pain, misery, and death. These attitudes permeated fictional representations of the disease: in a study of cancer in the movies from 1939 to 2012, an Italian sociologist found universal pessimism, with characters with cancer nearly always dying at the end of the story. I've come face to face with the immediate association of cancer with death many times during my life: Once, after revealing my occupation to a stranger in a pub in England, he shrank from me like Dracula from a crucifix. "Oh, you're Doctor Death," he hissed.

Doctors were not immune to these broader societal attitudes. How could they dare utter a word that is synonymous with death? Besides, cancer's mysteriousness and unpredictability were a rebuke to the new prestige and authority built on conquering infections. The association with death brought up feelings of helplessness and failure that were at odds with the heroic, optimistic narrative of twentieth-century medicine. Even when doctors did face cancer head on, there was still ambivalence – as shown in the naming of cancer clinics. In response to the rising threat of cancer, in the early twentieth century governments all over the world borrowed from successful strategies against infectious disease to create programs of "cancer control." "Cancer clinics," specialized facilities for assessment and treatment, were the centrepiece of these programs. Many medical experts were concerned that putting the word "cancer" on the signs outside these buildings would frighten patients away. In the 1930s, the members of the Cody Commission, the government commission set up to investigate and recommend the organization of cancer services in Ontario, Canada, prevaricated in the naming of Ontario's first cancer clinics and called them by the grandiose title "Institutes of Radiotherapy." It took many years for them to be renamed "cancer clinics." Hesitancy lives on today: many hospital cancer departments are known by the less threatening name of "oncology clinic."

The history of cancer has a parallel to the history of homosexuality, where a similar vocabulary of evasiveness existed until recently. Gay men are called "friends of Dorothy," their lovers, "companions." Lord Alfred Douglas, Oscar Wilde's lover, famously referred to homosexuality as "the love that dare not speak its name." In medicine, cancer is the disease that dare not speak its name.

From the start of my career, I witnessed such evasion. It was not uncommon for a new patient to arrive without ever having been told directly that she or he has cancer. All too often - as in Sam's case - the referring doctor receives the biopsy report and asks a secretary to book an appointment with a surgeon or oncologist without discussing the reason with the patient. It's incredible to me that a patient can be given an appointment with an oncologist, follow signs into a building marked "Cancer Centre," and finally sit across from me, with my badge displaying "oncologist," without fully understanding the reason he or she is there. And yet it happens time and time again. It becomes my job to break the bad news. Every time, I still have to take a deep breath before I emit the C-word, otherwise it catches in my throat like a fishbone. My facial muscles tighten into a defensive mask as if to protect me from an assault. It takes a seemingly superhuman effort to resist the temptation to resort to a bland word like "growth."

Prejudices rooted in history do not entirely explain the persistence of dodging and weaving around cancer. If I'd confronted the professor about his use of "trouble," he'd probably have muttered something about the need to be kind to patients and to avoid causing distress. He might also have invoked an old idea that telling patients they have cancer makes them give up hope and succumb more quickly. Families too often use this as an excuse not to disclose a diagnosis of cancer to a parent.

I suspect the real reason is more self-serving: to avoid the doctor's own distress. A frank disclosure of cancer can ignite anger, especially when there have been delays or mistakes in the path to diagnosis, or, as in Sam's case, previous doctors have not revealed the truth. Anger is often projected onto the bearer of bad news. There's also bewilderment: How could this happen to me, when I've lived a clean life? Obfuscation is a way of avoiding these unpleasant reactions and difficult, unanswerable questions – put simply, of just making the doctor's day go better. Its distasteful side is giving a false aura of lightness and optimism to an illness that even in its mildest forms can be challenging, both for patients and doctors. How much easier it seems to parry with a "shadow" or a "swelling" than with cancer.

But we doctors should know better. There is no evidence that the truth makes cancer patients more depressed, or that it somehow makes the cancer more aggressive. Evasion simply leads to confusion, anxiety – and mistrust. If the doctor can lie to me about this, what else might she be concealing from me?

Besides, the prevailing pessimism about cancer has no grounding in reality. My summer student experience showed me the truth: while many patients with cancer are diagnosed at an advanced stage and die, many others are cured. In between are a whole raft of patients with slow-growing cancers who live in symbiosis with the disease for many years. Statistics show that at least 50 per cent of all cancer patients entering a radiotherapy department can expect to be cured. For some diseases, such as breast cancer, it's higher; for others, such as lung cancer, it's lower. To some extent, the curability depends on the accessibility of the cancer to detection: because the lungs are hidden and voluminous, it's easy for a cancer to grow large before it's detected. A cancer on the lip will be noticed almost immediately and treated when it's small. But compared to other treatments, 50 per cent is a good average. Despite their more prominent position on the medical stage, my internal medicine colleagues in fields such as cardiology or endocrinology can't claim to really cure patients of coronary artery disease or diabetes. They can rearrange vascular plumbing or fiddle with the body's chemistry through drugs, but they can't eradicate disease completely the way radiation can. Despite decades of publicity campaigns by cancer advocacy organizations, much more needs to be done to promote the positive outcomes of cancer treatment.

Finally, evasion around cancer is connected to one of doctors' least-flattering attributes: a tendency to patronize patients, to regard them as easily fooled simpletons who can't handle the truth. Pussyfooting doesn't acknowledge patients' innate curiosity and intelligence – something the world-renowned Canadian radiation oncologist Dr. Vera Peters constantly reminded her colleagues about. "Patients are our best teachers," she wrote.

So it was with Sam. On the night before his surgery, as I'm leaving the hospital, I drop into his room. I tell myself it's to wish him good luck the next morning, but it's really to make sure my earlier fumbling hadn't upset him in some way.

The room is dark. He's alone, lying in bed, gazing at the TV screen, its reflections flickering on his face.

As soon as he sees me, he sits up, yanks off his earphones, and gives me his signature sunny smile.

"Hey, doc. Sorry about earlier. Sylvia's just worried."

"That's okay. Did Jeff come by and explain things?"

"Nope. Haven't seen anyone since you were here."

He looks at me with the precise gaze he must use when guiding a jet to landing.

"She's right, though. It is cancer, isn't it?"

There. He's said it. I freeze. My heart thuds in my chest.

Then as I slowly exhale, I relax. He's let me off the hook. He's helped me. The truth is out.

I meet his gaze down the same precise vector.

"Yes," I say, surprised at the newfound firmness in my voice.

He turns away and looks out the window into the small dark courtyard beyond. He presses his lips together. His eyes glisten. After a moment, he turns back.

"I knew it. Right from the moment you guys came in here with the long faces this morning. Do you think it's very advanced?"

"I hope not. That's why Dr. McCutcheon wants to operate. Surgery will determine whether it has spread."

He suddenly sits bolt upright and folds his legs into the same cross-legged pose he had at our first visit the day before. It's as though the truth energizes him.

"Okay, let's get on with it."

3

The Frightened Patient

With my father too, it's the patient who breaks the silence.

"Is it very bad?" my mother asks.

"Of course it's bad," my father snaps. "It's bloody cancer."

A log shifts on the fire, sending a brilliant flume of sparks up the chimney. Tessie rouses, scampers to a safer corner of the carpet, and collapses again in slumber.

The C-word uttered, the closet door flung open, I take a big breath and sink back in my chair. I tuck the reports back in the envelope and slip into my comfortable role of upbeat oncologist talking to a newly diagnosed patient. The script flows easily:

"If you're going to have cancer, prostate's the one to have!"

I sound like a used-car salesman trying to offload a defective vehicle. My God, is this how I sound to my patients?

"I was sure it was prostate," says my mother. "He's had trouble peeing for months. He wouldn't see anyone about it."

My father squirms and looks deep into the coals, embarrassed by this public mention of his urinary function. Like most men, he doesn't want to be reminded of the prostate – a tiny organ, tucked away in a dark place deep in the narrow funnel of the pelvis, the source of shame for its association with both sexual pleasure and, because it is so often the site of cancer, pain and death.

"The doctor in Calgary said he needs to go on those dreadful hormone treatments," my mother says.

"Yes," I nod. "The good thing about prostate cancer is it's very hormone sensitive. It can be kept under control for a long time with that."

"See, Russell. You must go through with it."

My mother's glasses mist with a film of tears.

"It's just awful, awful. He's only just retired."

I pre-empt uncomfortable questions about his future by climbing to the safe ground of my area of special expertise. Palliative radiation will shrink those deposits in his spine and ease his pain.

"I think the priority right now is for you to get some radiation."

My father frowns.

"It will help your pain."

He grimaces and emits a disgusted grunt.

I'm unexpectedly hurt by this rebuke of my chosen field. It's the strongest response to date of my decision to become a radiation oncologist. When I first told him, he muttered something about it being "interesting." I didn't know whether he was referring to my decision or the field.

If my experience with other doctors is any guide, he probably doesn't know much about it. Like cancer, radiation therapy is shrouded in mystery and secrecy. Medical students receive next to no exposure to it, so doctors enter practice with sometimes stunning ignorance of its uses. For most, it's a dark, closeted specialty, carried out in the dark dungeons of hospitals. My father's attitude is likely also coloured by his training in post-war London, when radiotherapy was relatively primitive, often carried out by cumbersome Deep-X-Ray machines that caused painful blistering of the skin.

Even at this early stage of my career, I've discovered one of the most onerous aspects of my job is convincing reluctant patients to undergo radiotherapy.

"I'm NOT having radiation!"

The old lady thumps her gnarled fist into the arm of her wheelchair.

Her name's Betty. She's a ninety-three-year-old artist and widow sent to me by a plastic surgeon, who's scrawled "SCC Scalp – for Radiation???" on the referral note. "SCC" is shorthand for "squamous cell carcinoma," a common type of skin cancer. Squamous, from the Latin *squama*, scale: under the microscope the cells resemble a disorderly heap of jagged scales shed by some reptile.

Betty's artistic flair shows in her poppy-coloured beret set at a jaunty angle on her head, blurry slashes of bright-red lipstick, and a pair of giant pink plastic hoops dangling from her ears. The only sign of infirmity is the wheelchair. One glance at her swollen joints tells me it's due to arthritis.

Her sixty-something daughter, Myrna, a younger, plumper version of Betty, with hair in tight, stainless-steel scrubber coils, stoops and speaks directly into her ear. "Mom, why don't you at least listen to what the doctor has to say?"

"He's got nothing to say that would interest me."

I indicate the note from the surgeon. "Dr. Feldman tells me you have a cancer on your scalp."

"I don't have cancer!"

Myrna's eyes swivel heavenward. "Mom. The doctor told you. He sent you here to talk about radiation."

"It's nothing. It's just a pimple."

"Pimple? You should see what's under that hat," says Myrna.

"Can I take a look?"

"Of course not. Myrna, take me home."

Myrna releases her hands from the wheelchair handles. "Absolutely not."

Time to turn on the charm. I lean forward and offer Betty a warm smile.

"So, tell me about your art."

She gives me a sideways look.

"Why would you care about that?" she says.

"She works in acrylics mostly," says Myrna. "Abstracts."

"Crazy stuff. I'm sure you wouldn't like it," says Betty.

"She's exhibited at international shows," says Myrna. "But the arthritis is making it more difficult for her to paint."

"Well, let me know when you have an exhibit. I'd love to see your work."

The corners of Betty's lips lift slightly.

"Myrna, get me out of here. We're wasting the doctor's time."

A glistening red streak appears just beneath the edge of Betty's beret. It slithers towards her right eyebrow.

"My," says Ivy, the perpetually upbeat nurse working with me, and immediately grabs a gauze pad from the cupboard. She dabs at Betty's forehead. Betty pushes her away.

"Will everyone just leave me alone?" says Betty.

"That's been happening more often," says Myrna.

"Can I take a look?" I say.

"No!"

"Mom. Let the doctor see. Please."

Betty gives Myrna a sharp look, then turns away, staring at the wall, as she allows Ivy to gently lift her beret. There's a dark wet stain on one side.

A blood-soaked wad of paper towel covers a large bulge on the right side of Betty's head. Ivy gingerly removes the homemade dressing, revealing what looks like a half-pound of raw hamburger meat plastered against Betty's scalp. Its craggy black surface is pocked with tiny craters filled with blood-tinged pus. Myrna steps back, hand over mouth, as the stench of rotting flesh floods the room. In their boundless growth, cancers quickly outstrip their blood supply, leaving their interiors, starved of blood, to rot.

A massive squamous cell carcinoma. It's obvious why the surgeon has sent her for radiation. To remove this tumour would require cutting off half of Betty's scalp and closing the wound with a skin graft from elsewhere on her body. That would be difficult even for a person half Betty's age.

"How long have you had this?" I ask.

"I have no idea."

Myrna's eyes swivel again. "A few years. We tried to get her to see a doctor, but she always refused."

"It's never bothered me."

"That's not true, Mom. You told me you were having pain."

Myrna explains that the odour and bleeding have stopped Betty from going out to her regular artists' circle meeting.

"You must miss that," says Ivy.

"At my age, what's any one going to do about this?"

I smile. "The oldest patient I ever treated for this condition was a hundred and five."

An image of Helena flashes in my mind. She was so scared I was going to write her off because of her age, she jumped up and performed toe-touches as soon as I entered the room.

"Compared to her, you're just a spring chicken. Can I check a few other things?" I ask.

I lean forward and run the tips of my fingers down the thin cords of the muscles of her neck, seeking any sign of enlarged lymph nodes that might indicate the cancer has spread. Betty shifts in her seat and the corners of her lips rise again.

"Well, I haven't had a man run his fingers over my neck in a long time."

"There's no obvious sign of spread," I say. "This is not going to take your life right now. You should consider some radiation."

"I already told you. I don't want it."

"What will happen if she doesn't do anything?" asks Myrna.

I explain that if the cancer is left to grow further, there's a risk of greater bleeding, infection, and more pain as the tumour infiltrates into nearby nerves and bone. Myrna's eyes widen and her steely bonnet fluffs out.

"We can't let any of that happen."

"Hah. I'll be long dead before."

"You look pretty healthy," I say. "A lot of fit people at your age live many more years. In the meantime, this will only get worse."

"What will radiation do?" asks Myrna.

I tell them it's doubtful it will completely eradicate a cancer of this size, but I'm confident it will shrink it.

"Did you hear that, Mom? Radiation will shrink it."

"And stop the bleeding," says Ivy. "No more paper-towel dressings."

"I just don't want it. Let's get out of here. Now."

I roll my stool back and stare at Betty. She glares back. I've witnessed patients' resistance before, but she wins the prize for obstinacy. Why doesn't she just take my advice? I'm the specialist, for God's sake. I'm supposed to know what's best.

I'm tempted to give up. After all, she's ninety-three, nearing the end of her life. I don't want her skin cancer to progress and kill her, but maybe that's what has to be.

People weren't always so reluctant around radiation. If Betty had her cancer a hundred years earlier, odds are she'd beg me to give it to her.

The discovery of X-rays by German physicist Wilhelm Roentgen in 1895, and of radioactivity by French scientist Henri Becquerel the following year, not only caused a complete revision of physics and chemistry, but also ushered in a period of radiation enthusiasm that lasted for almost half a century. The public was fascinated by the properties of these new entities. Individuals flocked to X-ray studios to have "portraits" taken, and X-ray machines suddenly appeared in children's shoe shops, purportedly to enhance the fitting of shoes. The luminous quality of radioactive materials led to a craze for radioactive dials on clocks and watches, radium-impregnated paintings that lent an ethereal glow to living rooms, and even radioactive face creams with the promise of eternally glowing complexions.

Doctors quickly seized on the medical applications of X-rays and radioactivity. For the first time in medical history, they had a tool that allowed them to see inside the living human body, and X-ray departments sprang up in hospitals everywhere. In addition, radiation had the obvious ability of affecting human tissue – a property discovered accidentally when

Henri Becquerel noticed inflammation on his skin beneath a pocket where he had placed some radium. If radiation could harm healthy tissue, it might destroy diseased tissue, and by the turn of the twentieth century experiments across the world showed that radiation did indeed have impressive healing powers. In an era when a doctor's therapeutic arsenal was limited, medical enthusiasm for radiation led to its use for all manner of conditions, from benign warts to goitres to tuberculosis. By 1902 X-ray therapy was so well established in medicine that three papers on its use appeared in one issue of the Canadian medical journal, the *Dominion Medical Monthly*. One doctor summarized the advantages of radiotherapy: "1. It is painless; 2. It leaves small scars, thus doing away with disfigurements; 3. It destroys diseased tissue, but not the normal; 4. It relieves pain; 5. It removes odour; 6. It removes the dread of an operation." This last advantage was particularly important in an era when the only treatment for cancer was drastic and disfiguring surgery. The introduction of radiotherapy heralded a promising new era of non-surgical treatment of cancer.

As radiation's medical benefits were being explored and trumpeted, its harms were slowly becoming apparent. Many of the early workers with X-rays and radium became "martyrs to radiation" when they suffered injury or death from its harmful effects. Marie Curie died from bone-marrow failure brought on by her lifetime exposure to radiation. In industry, the case of the luminous dial painters of New Jersey, who suffered painful necrosis of the jaw after licking brushes impregnated with radium-containing paint, provided a sad illustration of radiation's insidious dark side.

Radiation enthusiasm blinded the early experimenters and the public to these harms, and hindered rapid progress on care and regulation. The tide of opinion did not turn fully until the end of World War II, when the dropping of the atomic bombs on Hiroshima and Nagasaki, and the associated images of charred landscapes and burned skin, brought widespread horror and revulsion at this, the cruellest, most destructive use of radiation. Since then, the proliferation of nuclear weapons and accidents such as at Chernobyl, Three Mile Island, and Fukushima have kept the dangers of radiation firmly in public view and coloured attitudes to its therapeutic use.

In medicine, the indiscriminate, even careless, use of radiation gave way to a more disciplined, focused approach in which radiotherapy was administered only by qualified specialists in hospital settings. Specialists such as Toronto's Gordon Richards laid the foundation for the new specialty of radiation oncology through research into the biological mechanisms, treatment techniques, and effectiveness of radiation therapy.

Despite its new scientific footing, the specialty carried the burden of negative associations – a burden I encounter every day in the clinic with patients such as Betty.

Myrna releases the brakes on Betty's wheelchair and starts to swivel her to the door.

I can't let go so easily. She has no idea of the suffering ahead if this cancer remains untreated – if, for example, it does burrow into the bone, or deeper yet, into the brain. And, truth be told, her obstinacy has stirred up my own. It's like she's lain down a gauntlet.

"Wait, wait." I say. "Can you tell me why you're so against it?'

"I saw what you people did to Harold. I don't want any part of that."

"Who's Harold?"

"Her husband," says Myrna. "He had lung cancer and got radiation. It gave him bad side effects and didn't do him any good."

Yes, the side effects of giving radiation to the chest for lung cancer can be bad, the main one being painful swallowing caused by inflammation of the oesophagus. It's temporary, but can make patients feel like they're swallowing broken glass.

"Sorry to hear that," I say. "But this is a completely different kind of cancer. And the type of radiation we use for skin cancer is very different. It doesn't penetrate very deeply, so people usually get through it easily. The main side effect is a reaction on the skin a bit like a sunburn."

"Ha. My sun-tanning days are long over," says Betty.

"Okay. So how many treatments would she need?" asks Myrna.

"If we want to give her the best chance of getting it shrunk down, be-tween twenty and thirty. I'll have to decide once we map the cancer out in more detail."

Now it's Myrna's turn to poke me with a sharp look. "Twenty or thirty? That long? I can't possibly bring her here that many times. Some people still have to work, you know."

"Is there anyone else could bring her?" asks Ivy.

"Are you kidding?" Myrna pushes Betty towards the door.

"Mom, let's get you home."

"Hold on," I say. "I have an idea."

Myrna swivels the chair back.

"I'm getting dizzy," shrieks Betty.

It's time to go off-protocol. There's an established radiation regimen called "0-7-21" in which three large radiation doses are spread over three weeks. The long interval between treatments permits healing of healthy tissue, thus minimizing side effects, and it's convenient for patients and families. It's long been used as a palliative treatment for patients with poor "performance status," whose overall condition precludes multiple daily treatments. Often, they're bed bound and in the last weeks of life. Betty isn't like that, and I'm concerned about giving three whopping doses to an elderly lady's skin. I decide to modify it by using a lower dose given once weekly over six weeks.

Some of my radiation colleagues might look askance at such fiddling with radiation doses. Some would have just dismissed Betty when she refused standard radiation. But this is the art of radiotherapy – being creative in response to a patient's circumstances, as long as the creativity is within the bounds of safety. Not everything in radiation oncology, in-deed in all medicine, can be done by the book. Historically, creativity was at the heart of radiotherapy, since the first practitioners of the new art, devoid of scientific understanding of its underlying mechanisms, prac-tised by trial and error.

"Once a week? I could manage that," says Myrna.

Ivy's fiddling with her badge tells me she's getting impatient. We've got other patients waiting. She leans forward with a warm smile.

"Betty. Why don't you try it? If at any point you feel it's too much, I'm sure Dr. Hayter will let you back out. Right?"

I don't like the idea of patients stopping radiation after a few treatments, but in the interests of moving things along, I smile and say, "Right."

Ivy's smile disarms Betty. She scans our faces.

"Really. I can stop any time I want?"

I nod.

"Okay. Let's try it. But only if the doctor promises to give me another of his neck massages," she says, with a coyly flirtatious smile.

A few days later, I slouch on a chair in the doctors' workroom as I dictate a patient report into the hospital transcription system. A figure appears at my shoulder. I look up and see Ann, the radiation therapist in charge of the treatment-planning area. Formerly called radiation technologists (or techs for short), radiation therapists are the professionals who carry out radiation treatments. She's a tall, outgoing woman whose cheerfulness is matched by a collection of brightly patterned skirts that she wears under her lab coat. Today there are bright red poppies. I can tell from her insistent stare that something's wrong, so I quickly finish my dictation and hang up.

"What's up?" I say.

"Your scalp's causing big trouble."

I scratch the top of my head like a monkey and give her an inane grin. "Is it?"

"I don't think we can get her through it. Can you come see?"

I follow Ann's swaying coat down the main corridor of the radiation centre. Halfway, she stops, turns, and cocks her head to one side.

"This radiation prescription. I've never heard of it. Once a week for six weeks?"

"It's the only way I could get her to agree."

"Hmmm. Well, you're the doctor," she says with a slight tone of sarcasm that barely conceals her suspicion of my wacky approach.

We continue through a swinging door marked "Sim One." I immediately spot Betty perched on the edge of a treatment couch, glaring at two junior therapists, Edward and Fern, both newly graduated youngsters in white tunics who cower in one corner like frightened Bobbsey twins.

"Sim" is shorthand for Simulator. This is the rehearsal hall for radiotherapy, the place where the planning of radiation treatment begins. It's part hardware shop, part medieval armoury, part dominatrix boudoir, its shelves crammed with brackets, clamps, straps, buckles, and other devices for restraining patients. Sledge-like devices with movable wings, from which protrude cup-shaped brackets, lean against the walls: these are "breast boards," which are used for positioning women who require radiation to the breast so that their arms are not in the way of the radiation beam. A series of inflatable supports, that, when pumped up, grip the limbs or torso firmly into position, hang on a rack. Deflated, they look like carcasses strung in an abattoir. An object resembling a cannonball stares from a shelf: it's a circular lump of lead that pops opens like a clamshell, swallowing the sensitive gonads of young men to protect their testes during radiation.

As barbaric as these implements look, they serve a very important purpose: immobilizing patients in stable, comfortable, and, above all, reproducible positions. Because radiation is usually given daily over several weeks, it's essential from the outset for patients to be put into fixed positions that can be reproduced from day to day. The stakes are high: an accidental shift of a few millimetres from day to day can result in under-dosing of the tumour or overdosing a healthy bystander organ.

To one side, there's a stainless-steel counter arrayed with glass jars containing blobs of pink dental wax that is used to create immobilization devices for the jaw. For a patient with a cancer on the lip, it's vital to keep the mouth open to avoid radiation hitting the mouth or opposite lip, so he or she must clench a wax "lollipop" – a chunk of wax formed around a tongue depressor – between his or her teeth.

On the counter, there's a pot of India ink and a heap of syringes, used to apply tiny tattoos to the patient's skin once the treatment position is determined. Patients are either horrified or elated to learn they must receive a tattoo in preparation for radiation. The elated ones – "I've always wanted a tattoo!" – are disappointed to discover it's no bigger than a pinhead, while the scared are relieved at its barely noticeable imprint. These marks are reference points for the transition from the Simulator to the treatment machine. They also become permanent stigmata of admission to the secret society of radiation patients and have a very useful future purpose: if a person requires additional radiation in the future, the tattoos allow delineation of the first radiation area to prevent potentially dangerous overlap and overdose by a second. Many times, I've been grateful to identify a patient's tattoos, sometimes faded and almost imperceptible, from treatment received years earlier so I can plan safe re-treatment.

The centrepiece of the Simulator is a CT-scanner, its tongue-like couch ready to slurp bodies into its gorge, where fine X-ray beams chop tissue into electronic morsels to be digested, processed, and regurgitated as images on distant computer screens. Then, in the quiet darkness of his or her office, the radiation oncologist can examine the images and delineate deep-seated tumours. The final treatment plan, including the arrangement and intensity of the radiation beams, will be determined from the outlines placed by the radiation oncologist.

Betty doesn't need such a complicated process. Her cancer is on the outside of the body, visible to the naked eye, and it can be delineated with equipment that's childishly simple, almost daft, in the context of the sophisticated technology around us: a ruler and a magic marker.

But she does need to be immobilized – very important, since she's coming once a week, and the long interval between treatments might lead to changes in position. Edward and Fern have made a "mask" for her – a fibreglass contraption like a goalie mask that, when attached to a board on the treatment couch, will keep her head stationary. It has big round holes for her eyes and mouth, and a larger hole on her scalp where the slimy red face of the cancer glares out.

By the time I get there, the twins have already tried twice to fasten the mask, but each time Betty's kicked up a fuss. She's squirmed, struggled, screamed, and pushed it off. The young therapists have retreated to one corner, where Edward cradles the mask in his arms like a headsman with a freshly decapitated head. A disgruntled Myrna stands at her mother's shoulder.

Betty sees me as I enter the room.

"You didn't tell me about this!" she shouts.

"He did tell us, Mom," says Myrna.

"It's torture!"

I approach her. "Can I take a look?"

"No, no, no. I'm not letting them put that thing on me again. Get me out of here."

Betty tries to jump off the table. Edward and Fern rush forward and grab her. Betty clutches her head and groans.

"What's happening, Mom?" says Myrna.

"This thing. It's throbbing like hell. Why can't someone just cut it off? Or better yet, cut my whole head off."

Ann steps forward and places a hand on Betty's shoulder.

"We're just trying to help you," she says softly. "Why don't you lie down?"

Betty sighs and flops back on the table. I move to her shoulder and stare down into her eyes.

"Would a painkiller help?" I ask.

"That's right, just dope me up."

"Mom, stop being impossible," says Myrna. "Of course it would."

Ann summons Ivy, who brings a painkiller and a cup of water. She lifts Betty up and gives her the pill with a sip of water.

"Why don't we leave you alone to give that a few minutes to work?" I say.

Out in the corridor, Ann places her hands on her hips and glares at me in mock anger. "Thanks to her, we're running way behind," she says, indicating the waiting room outside the Sim, where three other patients perch in blue gowns. One of them, a white-haired man fidgeting with the ties on his gown, gives us a hostile glare.

"How much longer?" he says.

Ann beams brightly. "You're next!" She turns back to me with another glare. "We're spending more time on your palliative case than on these curable ones."

She's right. It's foolish to spend so much time and energy on someone who's being dragged kicking and screaming into radiation. Maybe I should just send Betty home.

Back in the Sim, Betty's eyes are closed. There's a soft snore that suggests she's sleeping.

"That pill knocked her out," says Myrna.

"Okay, quick," says Ann, and signals to Edward to replace the mask over her face. He lowers it slowly as if afraid of being bitten.

As Edward starts to pin the mask down, Betty wakes, grabs his wrists and pushes him away.

"No, no, no," she shouts.

They engage in a tug of war. The mask pumps up and down.

Ann grabs the mask. "We can't spend any more time on this today," she says. "Back to the drawing board, Dr. Hayter."

The usually timid Fern, a tiny girl with thick glasses, suddenly pipes up.

"Can I try something?"

"What's that?" says Ann.

"I can see where the mask is cutting into her chin."

Ann's and my gaze drop to the lower part of the mask, where yes, a ragged edge of fibreglass juts out. Good for Fern.

"Can I trim it a bit?" says Fern.

She pulls a giant pair of scissors from a drawer.

"Holy. What now?" says Myrna.

Fern snips at the mask, trimming away slivers of fibreglass, which flutter to the floor.

"Can I try one more time?" she asks Betty.

Betty looks at the refashioned mask suspiciously.

"Okay. Give it one more go, Mom," says Myrna.

Fern lowers the mask onto Betty's face. "Better?"

"Oh. Yes. Is it on? I can barely feel it"

"Thank God," says Myrna.

"Trust a woman to figure it out! Why didn't you cut it better in the first place?" says Betty, glaring at Edward, whose face turns crimson.

"Won't it be too loose?" I whisper to Ann.

"Better a bit loose than so tight she won't wear it," she says.

"Now there's one last step," says Ann. "Dr. Hayter needs to mark out the treatment area."

"How's he going to do that?"

Ann produces a magic marker from her pocket. Betty's eyes widen.

"Time for a little art!" says Ann.

"Make it quick," she whispers as she hands me the marker.

I go to the head of the bed, and come face to face with the nasty reptile, the corrugated, glistening *squame*, poking its head through the top of the mask. As if nervous of disturbing it, I gingerly feel round its edges with my left index finger, probing for subtle signs of insinuation under the skin beyond its visible edges. My right hand follows slowly, drawing a line with the marker around the tumour and any areas where I suspect infiltration. As I do so, I breath in a heady cocktail of solvent fumes from the marker and the pungent odour of rotting flesh. Betty is quiet, immobile, sleeping. Her rhythmical, sonorous breaths are a counterpoint to the low steady hum of electrical current coursing through cables in the walls.

Like spectators at a ceremony, Myrna, Ann, Edward, and Fern stand in a circle around me, their eyes fixed on the thin black line that appears from the end of the marker. I'm a sorcerer tracing a magic circle in front of an assemblage of priests. Yes, a *magic* marker.

Finally, the circle is joined, and I stand back to review my work. Oops, I can see in one area the line is much too close to the *squame*. I redraw that area with a more generous margin, then stand back and review once more. This time, I'm satisfied. The tumour, now encircled by a thick black ring, looks like a monstrous wrinkled eyelid circled by black eye liner. The sorcerer's work is done. I've created the target: the magic circle to summon and focus the destructive power of radiation.

Betty's eyes flutter open and she catches me staring at my work, marker still poised in one hand. Through the aperture in the mask around her mouth, I glimpse a smile.

"I know that look. I get it just after I've drawn something," she says.

A few days later, Betty returns for her first session on the "linac" – medical shorthand for linear accelerator. Strapped in the mask, lying on the treatment couch beneath its massive T-Rex-like jaws, she looks puny. When the machine is turned on, a surge of electricity will accelerate a beam of raw electrons deep in its belly, electrons that will eventually spew from its gorge onto the target on Betty's scalp. From among the various radiation modalities available, I've chosen electrons to treat Betty's cancer because of their limited penetration below the surface of the skin. After entering the tissue, they quickly stutter to a halt, dispersing their energy where it's most needed, in the centre of the tumour, thus avoiding damage to the delicate brain tissue beneath the skull.

The first treatment does not go well. It should only take a minute for the machine to deliver the required belch of electrons, but Betty keeps interrupting the treatment by signalling to the therapists, watching her on a monitor outside, that she needs a break.

After ten seconds: "Why's it so dark in here?"

Twenty seconds: "What's that sound?"

Thirty: "I'm freezing."

Forty: "I need a break! Take this damn thing off."

At each break, the cheerful, patient therapists switch off the machine and enter the room to explain, reassure, readjust, and comfort. A minute stretches to nearly half an hour.

At last it's over. As she's wheeled out of the treatment room, she glares at Myrna, sitting patiently nearby.

"I'm never going through that again!" she announces for the whole waiting room to hear.

I can't resist relief that today may be the last time I see her.

But it's not. About four or five days after the first treatment there's a noticeable improvement in her tumour. The pain lessens, and there's much less bleeding. Myrna convinces her to return.

I examine her before the second treatment, and yes, the reptile is already reacting: it's flatter, drier, less angry.

She goes for her second treatment, then a third, and a fourth. At each visit, the *squame* shows signs of collapsing and dying. The foul stench subsides. By the fifth treatment, it's retracted so much I have to redraw the margin of the radiation area to make it smaller. By the sixth and final treatment, it's withered to a flat dry scab, a flaky grey ghost of its former self. And apart from some redness and itchiness of the surrounding skin, easily dealt with by a simple salve, there have been no side effects.

The response of a tumour like Betty's always reignites the wonder I felt as a student when I witnessed the results of treatments such as the "Elastoplast mould" – the radioactive bandage applied to the patient's hand. The disappearance of an external cancer through application of a stealthy, invisible force always seems magical and almost miraculous. As I witness this process, I feel a deep connection to those pioneer radiation doctors who first applied radiation to skin cancers around the turn of the twentieth century and whose wonder and amazement stimulated research of this new modality.

As the tumour improves, so does Betty's attitude. On week three, she arrives an hour early for her appointment. Joking with her fellow patients about looking forward to her weekly "zap," she brings energy and humour to the usually quiet and sombre waiting room. She gets to know her therapists on a first-name basis and, as they fasten the mask on, makes small talk about their health and families. At her final visit she brings them a flowery thank-you card and a huge box of chocolates.

"Bye, guys! I'll miss you!" she chortles, as she is wheeled out of the treatment room for the last time.

A month after her final treatment, Myrna wheels Betty in to see me for a check-up. As at her first visit, she's all dolled up: She sports a brand-new tangerine-coloured beret with matching orange ear hoops. Strings of amber beads dangle across her chest. She looks relaxed and ready to take on the world.

"How are you doing?" I ask.

"You tell me! Take a look!"

She whips off the beret. Ivy and I take a step forward. We almost can't believe our eyes. The *squame* is gone, replaced by a zone of fresh, pink, hairless skin.

"Wow," says Ivy.

"Wow indeed," I say, running my finger over the smooth, baby-like skin. It's the best response I've had to date with my once-weekly recipe. I determine to offer it more often.

"Will her hair grow back?" asks Myrna.

"Sorry, unlikely," I say.

"I don't care about that," says Betty. "I'm just glad to be rid of that smelly old thing."

I summon Ann, Edward, Fern. Radiation therapists are not usually involved in check-ups after treatment, but I like to give them the chance to see the final results of their careful, patient handiwork. I also want them to see the results of my seemingly wacky approach. Smiling, eyes bulging in excitement, murmuring syllables of approval, they circle round Betty's head like space probes surveying a newly discovered planet. It feels like someone should pop champagne and toss streamers.

"We'll have to use this on more patients," proclaims Ann. "Once a week takes a load off the other machines."

Betty indicates a shopping bag hanging from the back of her wheelchair. "Show it to them."

Myrna pulls a large object from the bag. It's Betty's radiation mask, taken home as a souvenir and now transformed into a gaudy work of art. She's painted big heart-shaped red lips around the mouth and thick black lines around the eyes. Sequins sparkle on the cheeks. Around the opening where her cancer once protruded, there's a glorious golden sunburst.

"This is going in my next show," she says.

"Wonderful," I say.

"Thanks for not giving up on me, doc. You know, I was just afraid. I needed that push. Make sure you push all your other patients so hard."

4

The Uncertain Doctor

My father raises his hand.

"Enough about cancer. It's Christmas, for God's sake. Time for bed."

He leans forward and struggles to raise himself from the chair. I stand and grab one arm.

"I can do it." He pushes my hand away.

Emitting a grunt, he lurches forward, unfolds himself with a wince, and hobbles out of the room.

"Don't forget your painkiller," my mother calls.

She stands, grabs my wrist, and pulls me close.

"I didn't want to ask in front of him. How long does he have?" she whispers to me.

Her grip squeezes the truth.

"The hormone therapy will keep the cancer quiet for a couple of years."

She pulls me closer.

"Then what?"

"Well, there's always new treatments in the pipeline," I say, dodging her meaning with a forced tone of cheeriness.

She emits a weary sigh and releases me.

"It's dreadful. All this worry is making my lupus act up."

I draw her close in a half-hug, then she turns and totters off down the corridor.

I switch off the Christmas lights, give the fire a final poke and climb the stairs to the front bedroom. Tessie wakes and pads lazily behind me.

I lie in bed, listening to the soft snores of my slumbering wife and the fierce Atlantic wind howling around the chimney, thinking about my father's situation. Suddenly, cancer is no longer something foreign, something that I read about in textbooks or journal articles, or that happens only to anonymous patients. Now it's part of my family, right here, under my roof, in my house. A chill sweeps over my body, and I draw the covers up to my ears. I burrow close to the unconscious, comforting form of my spouse.

Not just cancer. Incurable cancer.

Yes, hormone therapy – suppression of testosterone, the male hormone that stimulates prostate cancer – will keep his cancer "under control," to use another sop, for a while. But eventually the malignant cells will regroup and thrash out stronger than ever.

Images of men with relapsed prostate cancer I've seen dance through my mind. The lean, athletic veterinarian with pain so severe, so intractable he begged to be put down like one of his sick animals. The big, strong firefighter who spent his final weeks in bed, paralysed and incontinent from cancer nibbling at his spinal cord. The medical colleague, a shy, spectacled pathologist, who became blind from a malignant deposit crushing his optic nerve. The friendly, outgoing insurance salesman whose legs bloated to replicas of whale carcasses from blobs of cancer obstructing the blood vessels. The kindly retired teacher who bled to death from invasion of his bone marrow by teeming hordes of cancer cells. As I slowly sink into sleep, my father's face, anxious and afraid, appears amid the teeming crowd of phantoms sweeping through my mind.

I don't wish any of these events on anyone, least of all my father. I want desperately for him to have time, time for us to spend together and forge a deeper connection.

But cancer is a nimble, cruel, remorseless foe who pays little heed to mortals' wishes.

~

At the end of a long day of seeing patients, I finish my last dictation, plop the Dictaphone receiver back in its cradle, lean back, stretch, then gather the patients' files into a bundle. I exit the clinic area and head towards the elevators in the cancer centre lobby. As I move through the crowd of departing staff bustling towards the revolving doors, a figure makes a bee-line towards me. It's Sherri, one of the dosimetrists, a radiation therapist with special training in creating radiation plans: maps of distribution of radiation dose that guide the placement of beams. She's a middle-aged woman with a kindly, cherubic face.

"Did you forget about Mr. Girvin?" she asks with a sly smile.

Girvin, Girvin. Which patient is that?

"You promised you'd have his contours back to me by the end of the day."

Of course. That short, burly Scottish guy I saw a couple of days back. Aircraft mechanic. Nicotine-stained fingers like they'd been dipped in mustard. A laugh that morphs into a deep, crackly cough. Yes, the one with advanced lung cancer.

"Oh sorry. Busy day. I haven't been able to get to it."

"He's booked to start treatment in two days. If I don't get the contours back by morning, I'll have to delay his treatment."

At his visit his wife unwrapped a tissue containing morsels of congealed blood. Somewhere during today's busy clinic Ivy had mentioned a call to say the bleeding was getting worse.

"No. I'll get right on it."

"Have a good night," Sherri says with a sweet smile and swivels towards the exit.

Poof. There goes my fantasy of going home and enjoying a glass of wine with Mark on the deck in the dusk. I swivel towards the coffee shop and pick up a cup of Earl Grey tea and a chocolate-chunk cookie to prime my brain with caffeine and sugar for the task ahead.

As the elevator glides up, I think: Sherri must wonder if I'm in cognitive decline. How could I not remember one of my own patients? But it happens all the time. In the whirling merry-go-round of the clinic, it's easy for a patient to drop off and get forgotten momentarily. It was nice of her to remind me so pleasantly.

At this time of day, the top floor, where the doctors' private offices are located, is eerily quiet. The administrative assistants' cubicles, usually a hive of activity, sit dark and empty. As I pad along the corridor, through half-open doors I spot a couple of colleagues tapping at their keyboards or poking at their phones. Knowing I have work to do, I don't stop to chat.

At one end of the corridor, Marcia, the cleaner, heaves the contents of a garbage bin into her cart. She greets me with a warm smile.

"Time to go home?" she says.

"Not yet," I say.

"You doctors work way too hard."

Her husband died last year of a heart attack. I give her a smile and a shrug, slip into my office and close the door.

Physical space in the hospital has not kept up with the growing medical staff. My "office" is actually a converted closet. Situated at the far end of a corridor, it's a small, windowless space lit by the pallid flickering glow of fluorescent strips. It's equipped with a desk, a file cabinet, and a bookcase, all fabricated from the dull grey steel typical of hospital office furnishings.

Still, this is my private space, my sanctuary, my refuge from the hubbub of the clinical spaces on the lower floors. I've added a few personal touches: my medical diplomas hang on the wall, their coats of arms staring down like escutcheons in a baronial hall, and my old medical school textbooks, including a dog-eared copy of *Grant's Atlas of Anatomy*, a greasy souvenir of hours in the dissection lab, line the bookshelf.

I've wedged a red-leather recliner, an impulse buy from a sale at a furniture store, in the space between the desk and the wall. Here, I occasionally have delicious secret lunchtime snoozes. Its presence has elicited an interesting range of responses from my colleagues, from sunny approval to sideways glances of jealousy, through to unguarded looks of reproach. My, my, a recliner? Aren't we supposed to be at work?

In between two of the diplomas, directly above my desk, there's a framed copy of *The Physician of the X-Rays*, a 1930s engraving by Austrian artist Ivo Saliger. It's a fanciful depiction of early twentieth-century radiation therapy and shows a portly doctor in a white coat and dark goggles at the controls of an X-ray apparatus that emits a stark white stream of rays towards a young female patient lying on a treatment table. In the foreground, the lanky figure of Death, a skeleton form shrouded in a black hood and cape, recoils from the rays with melodramatic revulsion – like Dracula recoiling from a crucifix. The young patient, caught in mid-startle at the rays' brilliance, sits up, crossing one arm over her eyes, a sunbather momentarily blinded by the sun's rays. The doctor is fully clothed, but the patient wears the flimsiest of sheets, revealing unabashedly voluptuous contours. The engraving is thought to be inspired by Saliger's sister's experience with cancer and radiation.

The image is an unsubtle and outmoded depiction of the gender and sexual dynamics of medicine, but I've always loved it. It alludes to scenes in classic horror movies, like the scene in *Frankenstein* where the monster is brought to life by electricity. More significantly, it's also an allegorical depiction of the essential drama of radiation oncology played out every day in the cancer centre: the struggle between doctors and death for the lives of their patients, with cancer being death's weapon, radiation the doctors'.

I set the tea and cookie on the desk, sit, and turn on the radio. The soothing tones of soft jazz fill the room. The leather recliner beckons, but I resist its seductive call. I send Mark a quick text telling him I'm delayed with an urgent case. He sends back a thumbs-up icon. I'm lucky to have such a patient guy in my life.

I turn on the computer, open the radiotherapy planning system, and scroll down the list of names. There he is: Girvin, Matthew. Sherri has planted a red flag by his name to indicate his case needs urgent attention.

I recall the details of his situation. Matthew's got inoperable lung cancer. A few weeks ago, he started to cough blood, and after his wife Muriel pressed him to get some tests, scans showed a tumour in his left lung. Biopsies confirmed a common form of lung cancer, squamous cell carcinoma. Those reptilian *squames* again: they sprout from almost every lining of the body. A surgeon declared his cancer inoperable, partly because it's twisted around several major blood vessels, and partly because Matthew's lung function is so poor he couldn't survive the removal of any lung tissue. He's been referred to me for treatment with radiation instead.

I click his name, and the system takes me to the CT scan images obtained in the Simulator. As in Betty's case, my job is to outline the target for radiation. But because Matthew's cancer is on the inside of his body, I can't use my magic-marker wand. Instead, I will use a little familiar, my computer mouse, to draw an electronic circle around his cancer. I'll also delineate his OARS – organs at risk, the healthy structures such as the heart and spinal cord, which must be spared from radiation. Once I'm done, I will forward these outlines to Sherri. Her expertise is creation of a treatment plan in which the radiation beams will be positioned and weighted to deliver a lethal dose of radiation to the Target Volume while at the same time limiting the dose to the OARS to a safe level.

Whether using a marker in the Simulator or a cursor in my office, the task of outlining the radiation target is the heart and soul of the technical aspect of my work. The later steps performed by dosimetrists and physicists all flow from this first essential step. It's why the staff sometimes kid me about being "the one earning the big bucks."

The task requires complete concentration and a steady hand. A wobble of even a few millimetres in my outline means the difference between cure and relapse, safety and toxicity. I close my eyes and let the mellow jazz calm my mind. I rotate my head to release the tension in my neck, take a big bite of cookie, and a swig of tea.

As the chocolate chunks dissolve in my mouth, I study Matthew's images to get a general idea of the extent of his cancer. I identify his "tracheo-bronchial tree" and follow its inverted outline from its roots in the throat, to the round, solid trunk of the windpipe, and down to where it splits into two main branches, the right and left main bronchi, which in turn divide and divide again into smaller and smaller bronchi, whose tiniest twigs eventually dissolve into the vast blackness of the lungs.

There it is: a grey, bloated, eyeless lizard, perched on the left main bronchus, folds of belly fat draped over the airway, its mass buckling the roof of the passage below, narrowing the air conduit. The stricture explains Matthew's harsh wheeze. Its spiny back curves into the nearby lung, and the tip of its tail brushes against the inner lining of the chest. Silvery claws reach centrally towards the heart as if searching for some foothold. In these static images, the creature looks dormant, but it's very much alive, pulsing, ravenous.

My God. The cancer is much bigger than I remember. I pull up Matthew's diagnostic images, the original scans done at the time of his diagnosis, and compare them with the recent planning pictures. Yes, over a matter of a couple of weeks, the cancer has enlarged. Its belly has swollen further to compress more lung tissue. Those silver claws grasp blood vessels. Worst of all, I spot a row of fresh grey eggs in the crooks of airways. I recognize them as enlarged lymph nodes, the first attempt by the creature to plant offspring outside its home territory.

I sit back and gaze at the screen. I told Matthew and his wife that I'd try to cure him but suddenly I'm not so sure any more. As a cancer gets bigger, and the number of cells rises from millions to billions to trillions, the chance of eradicating every last cell gets smaller. Even if we blast this creature with 6000 units of radiation – the standard curative dose for lung cancer – the chance of destroying it permanently is well under 10 per cent, probably less than 5 per cent. Plus, firing that much radiation into his chest is dangerous. Like the surgeon, I'm concerned about Matthew's lung capacity: to kill this cancer, radiation will need to pass through healthy lung, scarring it, rendering it useless. Even if he survives his cancer, Matthew might need to lug around oxygen tanks for the rest of his life because of what I do to him.

Maybe I should back off and give him a one-week course of palliative radiation. It will relieve his symptoms such as bleeding and cough – but give him zero chance of cure. A week of radiation will cause minimal side effects and can be done with a simple radiation technique that carries very little risk of permanent damage. In any case, permanent damage is irrelevant for someone who's going to die soon. He won't live long enough to experience it.

But this will be a major change in the goal of treatment. I'll have to recall Matthew and his wife Muriel for a difficult conversation. I'll have to explain his cancer has won: curative treatment is no longer possible, and the goal of treatment has changed from cure to relief of symptoms. I anticipate a discussion fraught with confusion, disappointment, and anger: Why the hell has the cancer been allowed to grow? Why wasn't this caught before? Why did you dupe me into thinking I could be cured? I'll have to tell him that he's now dying of lung cancer, and that his lifespan is likely less than a year.

At the top of the screen there's a banner with two boxes, one labelled Curative, the other Palliative. It's my job to signal my intent to the staff by placing an X in one of the boxes. Before I can start work on defining the target, it's important to mark one of the boxes. There's a vast difference in workload and impact on resources between the two approaches. A Curative plan requires hours of complicated mapping, calculation, and analysis, and a six-week booking on a treatment machine. A Palliative plan involves a simple radiation technique, usually what's called a POP (parallel opposed pair), where two radiation beams, crudely encompassing the diseased area, are simply fired at each other from opposite sides of the body. Palliative treatments can be arranged in a few days, sometimes hours.

Up to now, Matthew's intent is Curative. Should I change my intent to Palliative, and just POP Matthew to an early grave? I place my cursor over the Palliative box – but I don't click yet.

This is the moment when, to use a cliché, the doctor plays God. Or rather, a puppeteer, controlling the strings of patients' lives. Like my childhood puppet theatre, my screen is a playhouse with me at the controls.

Those two boxes become the familiar masks on the proscenium: Comedy, happy ending; Tragedy, sad ending. What will Matthew's story be?

On one level, Palliative would make my evening go better, since outlining a palliative target is far simpler than the painstaking task of drawing detailed contours around every millimetre of cancer and the OARS. Wouldn't it be nice to wrap up my work quickly, go home, and have that glass of wine before night falls?

My cursor wobbles. Despite the freshly laid eggs, there's no sign the cancer has spread further. Maybe I should give Matthew that 10 per cent chance. Maybe there's a way to deliver radiation while sparing normal lung. Radiation therapists like Sherri often come up with creative designs for radiation plans that minimize the dose to healthy tissue. And Charles! Your personal needs should not enter into the decision.

I wish there was someone beside me to discuss the case with, but the silence on the upper floor tells me my colleagues have long gone home. I hate to bother any of them at home. I could wait until tomorrow, but that will delay the start of Sherri's work.

Sitting alone in my dark, quiet cubbyhole, I miss the days when radiation planning was a more social affair. Prior to the advent of CT-Simulation and computerized planning, radiation oncologists marked internal radiation targets on ordinary X-ray films taken with the patient in their treatment position. We'd use information from diagnostic scans, from physical examination, and from basic anatomy to reconstruct the cancer, then sketch it on the films using wax crayons. It required an adeptness at a now neglected medical skill: surface anatomy, the delineation of interior organs based on external physical landmarks.

If you visited a radiation workroom in the early days of my career, you would have seen doctors clutching crayons and rulers, peering closely at X-rays, faces dappled with silvery shadows of patients' images pinned to the view boxes. They'd consider where to place their marks, draw, reconsider, erase, and reconsider again. They'd consult with their colleagues: "Am I missing a bit of tumour here?" or "Do you think this margin is too close?" And they'd deliver warnings: "Oh, watch out for that kidney." As the work progressed, there'd be chat about families and vacation, and hospital gossip, usually about some puffed-up administrator and his or her latest scheme for ill-conceived improvements. The radiation workroom had the lively, casual atmosphere of an artists' atelier. One of my mentors, Dr. Vera Kraus, a larger-than-life Hungarian woman, a lover of opera who could herself have been a Verdi character, chortled "Rrradioteraaapy – eet ees un arrt!" as she touched up one of her masterworks with a red crayon before sending it to the dosimetrists.

The process sounds crude by today's standards, but it had one advantage: because there was always some doubt about the exact extent of cancer, the margins of the target were always generous. In this way, "geographic miss" was avoided – a miss of the target by the radiation beams. These days, thanks to the detailed images provided by the CT-Simulator, we can place very narrow margins around our targets, allowing the use of high radiation doses unthinkable in earlier eras. But this precision comes with the risk of a geographic miss caused by miniscule shifts in a patient's position or a cancer's enlargement. The term "geographic miss" always evokes for me an uncomfortable image from an era when radiation oncology, like all of medicine, was dominated by men: whenever Bill Rider, an irascible Canadian radiation oncologist of the mid-twentieth century, referred to "Geographic Miss" in a slide presentation, he'd flash an image of a scantily clad woman draped in a flag.

Now, like me tonight, radiation oncologists are lonely puppeteers who sit by themselves in their dark, silent offices, gazing into flickering computer screens, pondering the fate of patients. Some of my colleagues do their work in an even more isolated way, from home offices.

Palliative or Curative? Tragedy or Comedy? A numbing wave of fatigue washes over me. Perhaps if I rest for a few minutes, my thoughts will become clear. I shift to the red recliner and push back. The soft plump leather envelops my shoulders, the leg rest cradles my legs. I close my eyes. The only sound is the soft whoosh of air in the building's air conditioning system.

"Why don't you let me take care of him?" a voice whispers.

I open my eyes and stare at the Saliger engraving. Death's face swivels towards me. His tiny eyes glint, steel bearings in black sockets.

"My, you look tired."

"I was wondering when you were going to pipe up," I say.

"Just tick Palliative and go home."

"I need time to think."

"About what? You know as well as I do he can't be cured."

"Sometimes there are surprisingly good results," I say.

"Bah. You and your puny radiation."

He flutters from the picture to the chair at my desk. As his robes collapse around him, the smell of damp earth fills the room. I sit up straight.

"Hey. What do you think you're doing?"

"You think you're the only one who's busy? I need a break too."

He reaches into one sleeve and pulls out a battered, heavily tarnished cigarette case. He thrusts it towards me.

"Smoke?"

"Of course not."

"It'll help you unwind."

"No."

"Suit yourself."

He pulls a cigarette from the case, fishes a box of matches from his sleeve, and removes a match.

"You can't do that here," I say.

"Rubbish. You know as well as I that people find places to smoke in here all the time."

There's a bright red flash as he strikes a match. My office fills with a pungent sulphurous odour. He lights up, takes a deep drag, and blows a stream of smoke in my direction. The sweet tobacco smell is strangely calming.

He shrugs. "I don't know why you're so surprised to see me. We've known each other a very long time."

"Yes. Drama. You're everywhere. Greek tragedies, Shakespeare, Victorian melodramas ... people die all the time."

"Bah! I've seen some of those. Silly fictions."

"I acted you once or twice in plays."

"Very badly, I may say. All that gaping and staring and gasping and pointing. Really. You know that I rarely make things so simple or dignified. Nothing replaces seeing me in the ... well, flesh."

"The cadavers in the medical lab."

"Those smelly things fished out of a tank? Hardly my best work. No. Don't you remember your shock the first time we came face to face?"

"That patient Sam?"

"We'll come to him later. No, before that. A nurse asked you to declare a patient dead."

"Oh, Mr. Baldwin."

"A stroke, I recall. I laid him out rather splendidly for you, didn't I? Arms flailed, mouth gaping. He reminded you of one of those petrified bodies from Pompeii."

"She coached me through it."

"Dear Grace." He takes a puff and smiles. "Poor thing, heart attack."

"Oh, no. She was so kind to me."

"'Honey, just check he don't have no heart sounds and no respirations, then put your John Henry right here.' But your hand was shaking."

"Yes. I was shocked and confused. This is a hospital; patients are supposed to get better. We can't just let someone die like this. What about his family? How will I explain this to them? And how will the doctor in charge take it when he finds out one of his patients has died? It was all so ... casual. The orderly came and bound his hands and feet together, and Grace stuffed his belongings into a plastic bag. They chatted about the weather."

"Mr. Baldwin was only the first. You discovered quickly that hospitals are just as much my domain as yours."

"I learned to cope. Nurses like Grace showed me how to make declaring death as routine as any other procedure."

"Routine? Oh, come on, be honest. I always do my best to add some variety, some spice. To keep you on your toes. And I always like to get under your skin. Leave a little reminder that the deceased was once a human being. The photos of children on the bedside table. The half-empty plate of homemade cookies."

There's a faint buzzing sound from something slung to a cord around his waist. He reaches into the folds of his gown, and pulls out an egg-shaped metallic object that looks like a hand grenade.

A screen on the device flickers to life, and he stares into it. His eyes glint, silver flames.

"Oh, dear. No rest for the weary." He stands. "Someone needs me on Ward 3B. Back to work."

As he stands up, his immense black shroud collapses around him again, this time emitting an odour of cigarette smoke.

"Just press that Palliative button. Leave the rest to me."

"Maybe I will."

"It'll make your evening go so much better."

The pager buzzes more insistently.

"Must run. I'll pop in to see how you're doing from time to time."

"Please don't."

He vanishes.

The buzzing continues. I open my eyes. The office is empty. Matthew's images flicker on the screen.

It's my phone. There's a text from Mark.

"U still at work?"

"Got bogged down with a case. Home soon."

I stand up, stretch, move back to the chair in front of the computer. The seat is icy cold.

I blink at the screen. Matthew's cancer glowers back. Yes, home soon. Okay, Palliative.

As I lower my finger, a ghostly image of Matthew's face appears in the murky grey fog of the computer screen. His eyes fix me with a look of intense desperation. Save me. Please save me.

There's something familiar about him. What is it? It seems like I know him from some place. Of course: my brother. How could I have missed that? My brother's also a fifty-something hearty British type with a zest for beer, rock music – and smokes.

Would I write off my brother? Of course not. Would I not give him the chance to live, however small?

I feel a surge of energy and sit up straight. What have I been thinking? I've got to give this fellow a chance. To hell with Death.

I tick Curative.

I take a swig of cold tea, grip the mouse, and start outlining. Click, click, click. Click, click, click. With each click, the cursor leaves a golden trail on the screen, a trail that connects to create another magic circle to summon the forces of destruction.

Thirty minutes later, I'm done. Lizard and its eggs lassoed in ropes of gold. I sit back and review my work. Wait, over here there's a small egg I've missed. Shit. I erase and redraw. And over there, a spiny outgrowth extends beyond my margin. I nudge the outline to include it. After a few more adjustments, I'm content.

Next, I snare the OARS within ropes of other colours – the heart in red, the healthy lung in blue, the oesophagus in pink, the spinal cord in purple. Click, click, click. These are circles of protection, of safety, guarding delicate tissues that must not be harmed.

By the time I'm done, almost an hour later, the screen dances with neon strings of colour, strings that circle and weave to make hoops and rings and ovals of various shapes and sizes. It has a certain prettiness, even flair.

But I'm far from finished. I've only drawn outlines on one slice. Matthew's cancer and his healthy organs extend upward and downward in his body for many centimetres, and so I must repeat the outlining on slices above and below the first one. I also repeat the outlining on scans taken at the extremes of inhalation and exhalation, since movement during breathing can affect the position of the cancer and the OARS. Through all this, I can't let my focus drop. I keep a firm grip on my sometimes twitchy mouse.

Finally, I'm completely done. I check my work one more time, make sure to save it, and forward it to Sherri. In the morning, it will be her job to design a radiation plan that ensures the heaviest dose of radiation lands in the circle of destruction, the lightest doses in the rings of safety. An experienced dosimetrist like her will know instinctively from one glance at my outlines how the beams should be oriented, how with a slight twist or change of angle of the beam, a touch of shielding here, a little more dose there, a safe and effective radiation can be produced. She'll use immense computing power to play with the radiation plan until she produces something akin to a weather map with "hot" areas in the cancer, "cold" areas outside. Her work, involving calculations, adjustments, and readjustments until a satisfactory plan is achieved, will take at least two days to complete.

I admire her talents and those of the other dosimetrists. Sometimes they're able to produce a safe radiation plan for anatomical situations where cancer and healthy tissue are impossibly entwined.

She's my fellow sorcerer. There's a special kind of wizardry in her work, wizardry I don't fully understand. I must trust her. Matthew must trust her.

5

The Disobedient Patient

We don't discuss my father's illness again during the Christmas visit. As he limps around, clutching chair backs for support and occasionally wincing, cancer remains an unseen, silent guest. At the airport I attempt to give him a hug, but he backs away, as if afraid my grip might worsen pain.

"I hope everything goes well," I say.

He grunts, turns, and hauls himself up the airplane steps. A few hours later, my parents are at home in Calgary.

During another autumn visit a few years earlier, I'm standing in their backyard, watching my father prepare the garden for winter. It's October, and the lawn is a dry ochre rectangle littered with dead leaves and twigs. A few withered brown stalks teeter in the flower beds. Through my jacket I feel the nip of cool air from the Rockies heralding the long prairie winter.

I watch as he methodically drags the rake over the lawn, creating even parallel strips free of debris. Then he turns and rakes strips of identical width at ninety degrees to the first. He puts the rake aside.

"Do you want any help?" I ask.

"No," he replies with a dismissive wave of the hand.

He crouches and sorts the raked harvest into piles of identical lengths. With a pair of shears, he cuts plastic sheets into strips corresponding to the size of each pile, then folds each pile inside a strip of plastic of the corresponding width. Finally, he binds each pile with lengths of twine.

My God, these are mere twigs. Why doesn't he just cram them into a garbage bag?

He allows me to help him carry the beautiful prepared bundles to the laneway behind, where he stacks them neatly against the fence. The final product is a cord of pristine plastic logs, so tidy and pretty that they must bewilder the garbage collectors.

My father did everything with such precision. He never crumpled a discarded piece of paper; rather, he creased it in the middle, tore it down the crease, turned the pieces sideways, and repeated until he had a collection of perfect white tiles that he laid carefully in the bottom of the waste basket. At the dinner table, he loaded each mouthful of food on his fork in the same order: first meat, then vegetable, then potato, finally a tiny dab of mustard, before placing the parcel in his mouth and chewing methodically. He once lectured me and my siblings on the correct number of chews to produce adequate digestion – was it thirty? Not: How was your day? How was school? But: Have you masticated sufficiently? Such it was to be a child in a medical family.

It must have taken extreme self-control and constant vigilance for my father to run his life this way. He was perpetually "wound up," as if a tight spring lay within him. A spring holding some shameful secrets in its grip. Even as a boy, I suspected one of the secrets was the cause of his parents' separation. For as long as I knew them, my paternal grandparents lived apart, in separate flats in the coastal towns of Hove and Worthing, England. They separated at some point after their arrival in England in the late 1940s and before my parents' marriage in 1950: the wedding photo shows them standing at opposite ends of the family group. There was a mysterious contrast between the expanse and comfort of my grandmother's flat, filled with treasures of ivory and brass from her life in India, and the shabby, cramped bed-sitting room occupied by my grandfather that suggested the acrimony of their separation. My father must have known the reasons, but he never spoke of it.

The other secret, which I confirmed long after my father's death through an analysis of my DNA, was his racial origins. Both of his parents were of Anglo-Indian ancestry – descendants of marriages between European men and Indian women. My research has shown that in the early days of British India, such liaisons were encouraged, but the tides of racism and colourism turned against their descendants – those of "mixed" or "dusky" race. My father bore the stigmata – black hair, brown eyes, full lips – of his family origins, but like others with the same background, did his best to hide it. Occasionally as a boy I witnessed vague and perplexing references to my father's ethnicity, such as when one of my mother's brothers noted my father had been "brushed with the tar-brush," or when my mother called him a "bloody half-breed" in one of her tirades.

On her deathbed, my mother revealed to me that one of my father's first acts after I was born was to inspect me for "signs."

"Signs of what?" I asked.

"The blood," she whispered.

He was scared his son's skin colour would betray his racial origins – I'll never know whether to protect the family from further shame or to protect me from bullying such as he may have encountered at his boarding school in England.

As a gay man who spent many years in the closet, I can relate to his constant self-vigilance and the pressures to conceal the truth. Perhaps too, my father's anxiety was born of his own need to measure up. His father was a decorated veteran of both world wars and a distinguished physician in colonial India whose career culminated in a glittering durbar at Government House in Calcutta, where, surrounded by serried ranks of Indian noblemen and a British guard of honour, he was made a Member of the Most Excellent Order of the British Empire (MBE). From what I know, my father had a lonely and neglected existence: he was raised by an ayah (nanny), then sent to boarding school in England – to him, a foreign country – at a young age. Like many boys raised in this style in this period, he had no consistent role model for a father – apart from the masters at boarding schools, of whom he spoke with warmth. After he arrived in England, an uncle befriended him and became a surrogate dad.

My father's precision and meticulousness, traits that today might be gathered under the rubric of OCD, must have made him an excellent doctor, but what effects did they have on the person? What toll did the daily self-flagellation and self-vigilance take? Was his cancer the body's final revolt against a lifetime of self-discipline? Did his cells rise up in rebellion? Doctors as prominent as Vera Peters have long ruminated about the possible effect of personality on the development of cancer – without, as yet, any firm scientific evidence.

Now, in the early weeks of 1989 after his cancer diagnosis, I wonder how he will cope with his illness. Will this man who has spent a lifetime controlling himself and his environment relinquish control to his physicians? Or will he, like some other equally intelligent, educated men I've encountered, try to chart his own course?

Early one evening in November, I'm summoned to the emergency room to see a cancer patient who's in trouble and might need urgent radiotherapy. As I make my way through the hospital, I glance outside and glimpse a few white flurries and dried leaves skimming and whirling over the asphalt, emitting brief flashes of white and gold against the blackness of late-autumn evening. Winter's on its way.

I wander through the twisting maze of the emergency department, where patients lie on stretchers or sit in wheelchairs, faces pale masks of anguish under the cold glare of the fluorescent light. My name tag dangling at my chest betrays my identity, and as I pass, patients and their families stir and watch me in an almost predatory way. Maybe that's the doctor finally coming to see me.

In one dark corner I spot a familiar figure. It's Death, leaning over a stretcher bearing an elderly woman, black robes falling across her torso, skeleton hand pressed on her cheek. He looks up, waves and smiles at me, then turns back to his work.

At last I locate my patient, Peter, a handsome patrician man of about seventy, with wavy white hair and shaggy eyebrows like frost-laden eaves. He's lying on a stretcher, propped up on a heap of pillows, within a curtained alcove. I immediately notice his pallor, his skin tone only one tint away from the stark white of the bed linens.

A younger man of perhaps forty with black curly hair sits on a chair beside the stretcher, holding Peter's hand. A son, perhaps?

One glance at Peter tells me he's in big trouble. A plastic tube bearing bright red blood emerges from beneath the sheets and ends in a drainage bag that slings udder-like on the stretcher's undercarriage. The bag is swollen with fresh blood.

"Hi. I'm Dr. Hayter, from the Radiotherapy Department."

He smiles and nods. "Good afternoon," he says to me in a raspy yet plummy English accent. "We've met before."

Oh, yes. Something about his accent and courtly manner strikes a chord of familiarity.

"You saw me about six years ago."

The younger man stiffens and looks at me.

"I told him to do what you said. But he wouldn't listen."

"You remember my husband, Carlo?" says Peter, shooting him an irritated glance.

Yes, I remember them both now. He's a world-renowned professor of architecture, originally from England, but settled and teaching in Canada for many years. The sight of him provokes an immediate nip of irritation.

When he first came to see me six years earlier, he had just been diagnosed with prostate cancer. For several months, he'd had typical symptoms, including a stop-and-start reduction in the flow of his urine. Carlo finally convinced him to see a doctor. He'd been found to have a tumour in his prostate, which on biopsy was an aggressive form of cancer. His prostate specific antigen (PSA) – a protein in the blood, an indirect measure of the extent of prostate cancer – was very high. (I saw Peter at a point in my career when PSA supplanted the acid phosphatase test used for my father.)

Peter's scans showed that (unlike my father's situation) there was no sign of cancer outside the prostate, so there was a possibility he could be cured. He'd been seen by a surgeon, who thought the cancer too large to be removed and referred him to me. When I first examined Peter, I found a golf-ball-size tumour in the prostate. The tip of my finger also felt tentacles of the primary cancer tethering it to surrounding tissues. The medical term for a cancer such as this is "locally advanced" – still localized to one part of the body, but extensive at its site of origin.

For such an advanced tumour, I recommended a double-barrelled approach: radiotherapy to the prostate, and a series of injections to lower the testosterone level in his body. Testosterone, the masculinizing hormone, is the chemical fuel for prostate cancer, and one way of attacking it is by removing this fuel. For locally advanced cancers such as Peter's, there was good evidence from published clinical trials that this approach worked better than radiotherapy alone. Although it didn't cure all patients, it offered their only hope of long-term survival. I had several men in identical circumstances who lived cancer-free for many years after this treatment.

As I explained my recommendations, he listened to me with his head cocked to one side, lips pressed in a slight smirk, as though he was listening to a paper by one of his graduate students.

"I thought that's what you'd tell me," he said.

He reached into a battered leather briefcase, pulled out a sheet of paper, and handed it to me.

"What do you think of this?"

Carlo, sitting at his side, emitted an annoyed grunt.

I glanced at the sheet. It was a list such as might be taken to a health-food store: vitamins C, D, and E, oils of flax seed and krill, extracts of turmeric, garlic, lycopene, milk thistle, saw palmetto, and stinging nettle. A veritable witches' brew of herbs and vegetable compounds.

Carlo peered at the list. "Did you include the green tea?" he said, roll-ing his eyes. "He has me brewing buckets of the stuff."

"This all seems pretty harmless," I said. "My only worry is the Vitamin C and E and the green tea during radiation. They're antioxidants, which can potentially reduce the effectiveness of the treatment."

Peter's lips curved into a caustic grin, as if he'd just tripped up a student.

"My good man, you misunderstand me. I want to do this *instead of* that awful radiation and hormones."

"Oh," I said. "Uh ... but you do understand that none of this will cure you?"

"Ah-hah! I knew you'd say that too."

He pulled a sheaf of papers from the briefcase and thrust them at me. I shuffled through them and saw they were printouts of pages from the Internet. I glimpsed headlines such as "The Secret Treatment for Prostate Cancer They Won't Tell You About," "Ten Herbs That Heal Your Prostate Cancer," and "The Cure for Cancer Is in Your Food." The shopping list was a cornucopia of ingredients he'd culled from these sites.

He leaned forward and stared at me.

"What do you think, doctor?"

I took a deep breath. "Well, this is all very ... er ... intriguing, but I don't know of any scientific studies showing any of this will get rid of your cancer."

"That's not what this doctor says."

He pulled out another sheet, a printout from the website of a Dr. Gomez in Milwaukee. Dr. Gomez's cherubic bespectacled face beamed brightly from a box in one corner. A quick scan showed the page to be an adver-tisement for Dr. Gomez's herbal cancer remedy, Prostacure, a concoction of many of the ingredients on Peter's shopping list.

"I'm sorry – I've never heard of this doctor or the remedy."

Peter shot me a haughty look full of surprise at my ignorance.

"Look down there."

The bottom of the page contained boxes filled with testimonials from prostate cancer patients who claimed to have been cured with

Dr. Gomez's remedy. Bill in Tulsa wrote, "I praise God every day for sending Dr. Gomez into my life. He gave me the cure I couldn't find elsewhere."

I handed the sheet back.

"You know, these are just anecdotes. My recommendations are based on clinical trials with hundreds of patients."

"You don't really believe they've been cured, do you?"

I took a big breath and decided to change tack. "Any idea how much this costs?"

"Twelve hundred dollars a month," Carlo said, swivelling his eyes again.

"Carlo, I told you already, there's a discount if I sign up for a year."

"It's a waste of money. Why don't you just do what this doctor says?"

Peter now turned his caustic grin on Carlo. "Darling, you do want me to be cured, don't you?"

It's estimated at least 50 per cent of cancer patients use some form of alternative or unconventional remedy, often including the herbs and vitamins on Peter's list.

There's a long history of alternative cancer remedies that runs parallel to the history of standard approaches such as radiation or chemotherapy. In the 1930s, Rene Caisse, a Canadian nurse, developed a herbal formula for cancer treatment based on an Indigenous recipe. She opened a clinic in Bracebridge, Ontario, which attracted cancer sufferers from all over the world. Never proven to help cancer, "Essiac" (Caisse's name spelled backward) is still sold as a laxative. A cursory search on the Internet reveals many other examples.

Why are patients drawn towards alternative and unproven remedies? Unlike Peter, many are in the last stages of cancer, desperately looking for something – anything – to give hope of recovery. Such desperation is often combined with denial of the truth. Many perceive alternative practitioners to be more patient and compassionate than regular doctors. Others are lured by the promise of gentle healing without the side effects of surgery or radiation. They are drawn towards so-called natural products, apparently innocuous substances derived from nature, different from toxic chemicals fashioned in the labs of giant pharmaceutical companies. According to this common notion, natural substances are innately beneficial; manufactured remedies, harmful. Such thinking lies behind the reluctance of many to receive vaccination during the COVID-19 pandemic.

A glance at medical history shows this distinction to be false. Many conventional Western medicines are derived from "natural" products – digitalis for heart failure from the foxglove plant, aspirin from willow bark, penicillin from mould, vaccines from inactivated viruses, and an early chemotherapy drug, vincristine, from the rosy periwinkle. Even radiotherapy can be considered "natural" – after all, humans are constantly bombarded with background radiation from the cosmos and the rocks underneath us. The first successful radiation treatments were given using radium, a naturally occurring radioisotope refined from pitchblende ore.

Conversely, "natural" remedies are not always innocuous. Some are adulterated with potentially harmful chemicals. Remedies for sleep and erectile dysfunction labelled as natural alternatives have been found to be laced with compounds that carry risks of side effects, allergic reactions, and interactions with prescription medicines. Some contain toxins such as lead or arsenic. Even compounds completely derived from natural sources are not without risks. Ginseng, for example, interacts with warfarin, a commonly used blood thinner.

For me, "regulated" and "unregulated" remedies is a more useful distinction. The production and distribution of regular medicines are controlled by standards that dictate their chemical composition and proof of their efficacy – standards enforceable by law. When you have a headache and take a 500 milligram acetaminophen tablet, you can be as sure as possible that is exactly what you're putting in your body, and there is background proof that it works. The composition of many so-called natural remedies is unregulated, and many have leap-frogged from idea to market, bypassing the intermediate phase of testing for proof of their efficacy. Patients take risks when they use them.

The history of my own field, radiotherapy, illustrates the dynamic boundary between unregulated and regulated treatments. Initially, radiotherapy was viewed with as much scepticism as Essiac. A 1914 editorial in the *Canadian Medical Association Journal* denounced the "new quackery" of radium. This attitude lingered well into my career: on learning of my decision to enter radiation oncology, an internist wondered aloud what on earth would make me interested in "hocus-pocus." As evidence of efficacy grew, radiotherapy slowly merged into the centre lanes of medicine, albeit in the blind spot of more glamorous drivers. Medical history is filled with similar examples of therapies and procedures moving from the fringes to the centre through an intermediate zone of laboratory experimentation and clinical trials.

As historians and sociologists have shown, many factors influence which therapies gain access to the laboratory and later, the market. I understand the political and economic biases – not the least of which is the influence of Big Pharma – that lie behind which compounds are chosen and submitted for testing and regulation, but I don't believe, as some activists have suggested over the years, that there is some huge conspiracy to withhold promising cancer treatments from the public. Believe me, oncologists would be delighted if a miracle cure emerged that allowed us to discard our often brutal triad of surgery, radiotherapy, and chemotherapy. In fact, oncologists' enthusiasm has sometimes led them to rush promising new treatments to the clinic before their true effectiveness or toxicity was completely understood.

A large proportion of patients keep their use of alternative remedies secret from their oncologists. Secrecy can be dangerous, since many natural products have biological effects, and, as in the case of Peter and his antioxidant vitamins, can interfere with the regular treatment. In recognition of the common use of alternative remedies and of concerns about safety, health organizations have recently tried to bridge the divide between regular and alternative practices. In 1992 the National Institutes of Health (US) established the Office of Alternative Medicine to facilitate the scientific study of alternative practices. This office is now known as the National Center for Complementary and Integrative Health. The title itself challenges the old antagonistic model of alternative and allopathic practitioners.

On the ground in the clinic, there have been attempts to foster collaboration. In a novel and brave initiative, the director of a cancer centre where I worked invited a local naturopathic physician to team up with me during a weekly clinic. We both started the association a little wary of each other, but with time, mistrust broke down and we learned from each other. When I saw that her approaches seemed helpful in easing side effects and lending patients a sense of control, I had to swallow some of my allopathic hubris. Such collaborations remain rare, and regular cooperation between allopathic and alternative clinicians remains an elusive dream.

At least Peter had been open with me about his plans. I recited my standard speech for patients interested in alternative remedies:

"Of course, you're free to explore any treatment you want. But it's my job to warn you about two things: There are lots of unscrupulous individuals out there looking to make money off cancer patients, so don't get involved in anything that might cause you financial hardship. And watch out for side effects."

"Money is no issue," said Peter. "And if I get some side effects from Prostacure, it will be nothing compared to radiation and hormones."

I told him yes, radiation would certainly have some short-term side effects such as diarrhoea and a burning sensation with urination, but these would go away within a week or two of finishing treatment. A small number of patients, less than 5 per cent, have long-term complications such as scarring of the urethra or rectum. And the typical side effects of hormone therapy would be hot flushes, tiredness, and loss of libido.

"Libido? We don't want that," Peter said, glancing at Carlo.

He tucked his notes back in his briefcase, snapped it shut, and rose.

"Thank you for your time, doctor. I'm glad we came to see you. It just confirmed my opinion I don't want anything to do with radiation or hormones."

My experience with patients such as Betty had taught me not to give up easily. It was time for me to get tough.

"Look. I'm not going to pull any punches. You have a bad cancer. Radiation and hormones is the only way of getting rid of it. Otherwise you could die."

He stared at me with the kind of stiff unyielding bulldog glare only the British can pull off. I forced a smile and stared back, inwardly wondering what caused this man's obstinacy. Usually conversations about alternative therapies ended in compromise: for example, a decision to use a complementary therapy alongside radiation, or wait and use it later. But this man wanted to walk away from a potentially life-saving treatment.

As I returned his stare, I suspected the underlying reason: control. Like many male patients I'd seen, including my father, with whom he shared some mannerisms, Peter was used to being in charge. He was now faced with the ultimate challenge: cancer, by definition, an uncontrolled and sometimes uncontrollable enemy. Instead of surrendering, cancer only forced him higher on the ramparts, where he stood now fully armed, sword drawn, eyes blazing.

Carlo stood and broke the silence. "Why don't you think about what the doctor says," he whispered.

"No," Peter barked. "Off to the health-food store for some shopping."

He turned and marched from the room. Carlo gave me an apologetic shrug then followed.

I strode to the workroom, tossed his file on the desk, collapsed in a chair, and emitted a groan. My heart thudded rapidly.

Ivy glanced at me from her desk. "You look upset," she said.

"That man didn't want to listen to a thing I had to say."

She smiled and handed me a cup of freshly made herbal tea.

"Don't let it bother you. He's a smart guy. You gave him his options. It's his life," said Ivy.

I agreed intellectually. But as I sipped the tea, I silently stewed in anger. I'd been conditioned by training that viewed patients as cases, not as human beings with wills of their own: patients as mere subjects of doctors' "orders." Doctors as puppeteers, controlling the strings of marionette patients. As a trainee, I'd witnessed encounters in which my teachers had explained treatments to patients hurriedly, with no opportunity for questioning or options. Later, I often overheard conversations between my colleagues and patients where treatment was offered as a fait accompli, with no suggestion there might be an alternative – especially one suggested by a patient. I'd seen my teachers and colleagues bristle with indignation when a patient dared to question their authority. I'd done my share of bristling – like now, in the aftermath of my encounter with Peter.

Patients like Peter were in the vanguard of those who wanted, even demanded, to snip their marionette strings and have a role in decisions about their treatment. The historical background was decades of public frustration with the medical establishment's arrogance, which culminated in activism in the areas of women's health and AIDS. The advent of the Internet, which empowered patients such as Peter with information, heralded the end of the paternalistic model. A patient armed with a binder full of information culled from Dr. Google started to become a familiar sight and forced me towards a new role: that of a teacher whose job is to guide patients through the copious and often conflicting information they've gathered and to offer recommendations, not orders, about the best course of action.

This more collaborative role was more time-consuming because it involved discussion rather than simply barking commands, but in time I found it more satisfying for me and my patients. I've always enjoyed teaching. Patients left the consulting room feeling they have played a part in decisions about their health, and I felt like they understood what they're facing. It was also a relief – I no longer bore all the responsibility for decisions. Mentally competent patients were free to accept or discard my advice – although, truth be told, there was always a slight sting when they rejected it.

As time went on, I became so accustomed to my new role that it was a surprise when I encountered, as I sometimes did, a patient who preferred the old style of doctoring. After I concluded with "So, these are your options. What do you think? Have you thought about what you'd like to do?" they would look at me in stunned surprise. "You're the doctor. You know best. I'll do whatever you say."

But my encounter with Peter occurred early enough in this transition that it was still a shock to meet a patient who so firmly wanted to chart his own course. Of course, as so often happened in my work, the nurse was right. It was Peter's life. As long as he was mentally competent, he could choose any treatment he wanted. And I had to face up to an ugly truth: Wasn't my anger a result of my own need for control?

Ivy's tea has soothed me. But one doubt remained: If I let Peter go untreated, am I not complicit in a death? Can I live with that?

I turned to her. "I'd better make damn sure this is what he wants. Can you book him to see me again in a week?"

He didn't show up for the second appointment. I called him and went through an abbreviated version of our first discussion. He told me firmly he hadn't changed his mind.

Over the next few weeks, I called him several more times and always got the same response. Over time, his replies grew shorter and snippier. Then the calls started to go to voice mail. I called his family doctor, who told me he rarely heard from Peter and wasn't even sure he was in the country.

Eventually, I had to give up. I'd done my best. I took a big breath, opened his file, and wrote a note documenting our conversation and his decision. I closed his case.

I thought the next I'd hear about him would be his obituary in the paper.

Now, here he is, six years later, in the emergency room, exsanguinating in his urine. Scans show his cancer has clawed its way into his bladder, where it's ripped great bleeding gashes. His PSA is over 2000, indicating his cancer has metastasized widely.

As I stand by his gurney, gazing at the stream of blood coursing into the drainage bag, I feel a strong urge to stomp my foot, wag my finger, and shout "I told you so! Why didn't you listen to me? That stupid Prostacure doesn't work!" If he'd gone along with my recommendations six years earlier, there's a good chance he wouldn't have ended up like this.

But I have to reign in my anger. There's no point in revisiting the past. At this point, he's in a dire situation and something must be done.

"We need to get you into the hospital and start some urgent radiation."

"Radiation? No, no."

"It's the only way to stop the bleeding. Otherwise you can bleed to death."

In the corner beyond the stretcher, Death twirls an exultant pirouette.

"Of course he'll do it," Carlo says. "No questions asked."

Death spins to a halt and frowns.

Carlo fires a stern look at Peter, who emits a melodramatic sigh and looks at the ceiling.

"All right. Get on with it."

As a porter shoves Peter's stretcher towards the radiation department, Death scurries away.

Within a couple of hours, Peter's received his first dose. A couple of days later, I pay him a visit. He's propped up in bed, scrawling in a notebook, pages of a manuscript scattered over the covers. His skin tone is now pink. The liquid sloshing in the drainage bag has turned from claret to rosé. He peers at me over the top of his spectacles.

"Was that machine turned on?"

"Why do you say that?"

"No side effects."

"Good. It's working. Your bleeding is slowing."

"Yes. I do feel better. Stronger."

He lays down the manuscript, drops his face, and looks up at me sheepishly through his eyebrows.

"I was stupid, wasn't I?"

"What do you mean?"

"That Prostacure was rubbish, just like you said."

"You did what you had to do."

"It's obviously not working any more. Are things very bad?" he says.

His new scans showed that the cancer had spread into the lymph nodes as well as his bones.

"Cripes. So I'm done for?"

I nod. "I'm sorry. It's not curable anymore."

The bulldog mask on his face melts, revealing a boyish, softer, more vulnerable face.

"Gosh. I'm not ready to die. I've got so many things I want to do. This is a chapter of a book I'm working on. And did I tell you I sing in a local opera society? They're doing *Pirates of Penzance* next fall. I had hoped to try out for the Major-General."

"Well, there's a bright spot. Your cancer is hormone naïve, meaning it's never been exposed to hormones, so there's a good chance even now it will respond. It's a bit like bacteria never exposed to antibiotics."

"Those hormones. Will I need to buy a bra?" He smiles and winks. "Maybe I'll branch out to drag. How much time will it buy me?"

"Two, maybe three years."

"That'll give me enough time to get this book out and do a show or two. Let's do it."

The mask hardens again.

"But if I find the side effects intolerable, I'll stop."

Over the next few days, Peter's bleeding completely stops, his drainage tube is removed, and he is discharged from hospital. Before he leaves, he's given his first injection of hormone therapy.

I see him a few weeks later. His cheeks are plump and red. His appetite and energy level are good. His PSA has plummeted, indicating his cancer has reacted well to the drugs.

Best news of all, he got the role of the Major-General. He arranges tickets for me and my partner Mark.

As we sit with Carlo, watching him prance on stage in a red uniform and feathered hat, rattling off the famous patter-song, a niggling thought arises. Six years? That was a long time for an unproven remedy. Was it luck? His iron will? Sheer determination?

Could it have been Prostacure? Ha. Like the early radium doubters, I'm starting to think: maybe there's something to it after all.

6

The Ornery Surgeon

After my parents return to Calgary, my mother keeps me informed through her favourite mode of communication: letters written on blue notepaper in her characteristically scrawled handwriting, t's crossed by loopy backward extensions of the last letter in each word, like billowing sails propelling the words towards the tilting horizon of the paper, shoving her favourite punctuation mark, the exclamation, overboard.

She tells me my father's seen a urologist, an ex-Brit with a hyphenated last name – my parents always deeply distrustful of anyone who trained outside the UK. He's booked my father for "that nasty procedure": a TURP – a transurethral resection of the prostate, basically, a reaming of swollen prostate tissue using a tiny rotor inserted in the urethra. How will my father, an intensely private man, suffer the indignity of lying on the operating table in full view of a gaggle of nurses as a miniature roto-rooter inserted up his penis whirs and chops his prostate into slivers that fall into a bucket between the urologist's legs? I understand the need for the procedure – to relieve his urinary symptoms – but I'm also worried it will create a delay in treatment of his overall condition. The cancer has long departed its home territory and established colonies in the bone that need to be brought under quick control.

My father survives, and the harvest from the prostate shows aggressive cancer cells. I become more worried when the urologist doesn't refer my father to an oncologist like me for further treatment. Instead, he

takes over treatment of the cancer. It's not surprising: in the territorial
division of the body, urologists "own" the prostate and its diseases, and
often manage patients with prostate cancer themselves. Often, they refer
patients to oncologists only when their remedies fail. The cynic in me
says he won't let go also because, in a fee-for-service system, he'll lose the
income from his patient. Resistances like this are the reason only a proportion of cancer patients are ever seen in cancer centres. I also suspect
it's my father's privacy: seeing the urologist in his private office spares
him the torment of walking into the public lobby of a cancer centre.

Since the 1940s, the mainstay of treatment for metastatic prostate
cancer has been "androgen ablation," the treatment I offered to Peter in
conjunction with radiation, which involves removing the cancer's supply
of the male sex hormone testosterone, on which it relies for its growth.
While not a cure, androgen ablation often produces impressive remis-
sions. The simplest method is removal of the testicles. I'm worried the surgeon's reflex reaction will be to castrate my father, or, if my father refuses,
to chemically castrate him with the female hormone estrogen. I envisage
my father as either one of those pale, depressed eunuchs I've seen in my
clinic or one of those men who develop plump breasts as a side effect of
estrogens and whose wives tease them with offers of loaning a bra. Ablation, yes, not just of the hormone but also of the *andros*, the male person.
As a resident I witnessed the use of preventive radiation to the breast area
to prevent enlargement in men about to embark on estrogens.

Castration or feminization will have devastating effects on my father's
psyche. I have several photos of him as a young man, one of which shows
him squatting on a beach in a bathing suit, displaying a slim, lithe, athletic body. He retained pride in his physique his whole life. From his
erect bearing – shoulders always thrust back, chest out – and from casual
remarks over the years I know that, like other men of his generation, he
has a firm mental image of the way men should look and behave. One
of the few times he spoke sharply to me as a boy was when he asked me
to loosen the hood of my duffel coat because he thought its tightness
accentuated girlish features.

I hope the urologist knows there are alternatives. Even before my father's illness, I had an interest in prostate cancer, kindled during my residency by Dr. Friar, one of my radiation oncology mentors. I'd kept up to date, and knew there were newer hormone manoeuvres that didn't produce the same drastic side effects as castration or female hormones. Some lowered testosterone by interrupting the signals the brain sends to the testes, others by blocking the entry of testosterone into cancer cells. In fact, in August 1989, just before the visit when I noticed my father's pain, a publication showed that "total androgen blockade" – the combination of a signal-interrupting injection with an oral testosterone blocker – was superior to the injection alone. These results sent a buzz through the oncology community, and androgen blockade became all the rage for treatment of metastatic prostate cancer. But has the buzz reached this independent surgeon's ears? Is he up to date? Or is he one of those conservative surgeons who stick to the "tried and true" – even though, as Vera Peters once said, the "tried" is not always "true."

My worries coalesce into a strong urge to play a role in my father's care. Maybe I should call the urologist and have a friendly chat to suss out his knowledge of prostate cancer, and if it's not up to snuff, to ask for my father to be referred to the local cancer centre.

"You know, just to cover all bases," I rehearse.

But I don't. Surgeons – particularly Brits with hyphenated last names – don't like non-surgeons questioning their decisions.

It's Friday at lunchtime, and I sit at a large rectangular table in a windowless conference room deep in the hospital's cancer centre, munching on a slab of cold pizza from a paper plate. The faint hubbub of the hospital corridor outside penetrates the heavy wood of the closed doors.

I'm at the Genitourinary Multidisciplinary Case Conference, a private weekly meeting of the specialists involved in treatment of patients with cancers of the genitourinary tract – the long conduit, essentially a sophisticated plumbing apparatus, that carries urine from the filtration plant of the kidneys down through a narrow pipe called the ureter into the bladder reservoir and, finally, to the outside via another pipe, the urethra – which, in a male, is sheathed inside the penis. In men, this tract also serves sexual and reproductive functions and includes the prostate (a small gland encircling the urethra where it exits the bladder) and the testes. The purpose of the meeting is to discuss cases and reach a consensus about the best treatment for the patients under discussion. There's a separate Gynecological Oncology Case Conference, which focuses on female cancers such as uterus, ovaries, and vagina, and similar weekly conferences for other cancer sites, such as breast, lung, and skin cancers.

Doctors face each other across the vast table. The non-surgical specialists, the radiation and medical oncologists, sit on one side, in drab lab coats, facial creases accentuated by the harsh overhead light. The surgeons, urologists, in rumpled operating-room greens, sit facing us. Representatives of the diagnostic specialties sit at the end: a thin female pathologist in cardigan and pearls, and a plump male radiologist in a striped golf shirt. As we await the start of the conference, there's no interaction: everyone hunches over their cell phones, and the room is silent except for the sounds of slurping and chomping on pizza and the occasional half-suppressed grunt or snort in response to a message or image on their screens.

Time was when attendance at such rounds was sparse. Doctors, always independent creatures, are downright allergic to disagreement, which often happens at these conferences. If they want advice, they prefer to corner a trusted colleague for a quiet discussion in a corridor. Somewhere along the way a bureaucrat overseeing the cancer system decided that there must be a multidisciplinary discussion about every new cancer case, no matter how trivial or routine. Participation was improved by incentives of free pizza and a small fee paid to each doctor for submission of cases. It's become a bit like grade school: there are careful attendance records summarized into statistical reports dutifully submitted back to the bureaucracy. Such records fail to mention whether the discussion was of any benefit to the patient. Showing up and making a tick mark to show a case was discussed is enough to keep the pizza boxes arriving.

Of course, not all discussions are pointless and useless to a patient's care. They provide an extra measure of assurance and support about important, potentially life-saving decisions. I've often benefitted from valuable new insights into a case provided by my colleagues. Possibly too, the record of a discussion mitigates an allegation of malpractice, since theoretically a group decision carries more weight than an individual one. Most cases discussed here, however, are routine, and the time would be better spent on truly perplexing cases for which the way forward is not easy for an individual doctor to decide.

Finally, the chair of the conference, the chief of urology, Dr. Little, strides into the room and scrawls his name on the sign-in sheet. He's a squat, pugnacious-looking man of about fifty with a crew cut and a flat, squashed nose suggestive of injuries from a previous boxing career. Like his fellow surgeons, he's clad in a set of wrinkled operating-room greens. A surgical mask hangs loosely beneath his chin and his operating-room cap is set at an oddly rakish angle.

"Sorry I'm late. Got tied up in the OR. Let's get started."

He grabs a slice of pizza and flips open a file folder.

"Okay, first case. Fifty-six-year-old fellow. Cancer of the penis."

The mostly male attendees squirm slightly in their seats.

"Usual story. Fellow noticed a lesion on the shaft a few months ago. GP messed around with liquid nitrogen. Didn't go away, sent him to me. I took a bite last week. Dr. Canning, let's look at the path."

"Bite" is surgeon-speak for a biopsy, a tissue sample.

The pathologist gathers her cardigan around her, goes to a podium, and fiddles with the controls. The room darkens, and a screen lights up. The doctors look up from their phones and gaze at the image: an irregular pink blob.

The reflected light from the screen transforms the darkened room to a study in red: the doctors' pale faces become rosy masks, Dr. Canning's pearls pulse like radioactive cherries, and crimson daubs of tomato paste glisten on the paper plates.

I make out the figure of Death, sitting at the back in the corner, his skull pink coral. He gives me a wink as he picks a scrap of tomato skin from between his craggy front teeth.

All eyes focus on the blob, a satellite image of an unknown continent, edges frayed by deep bays and jutting peninsulas, interior dotted with pools and rivers. A map, or maybe a piece of abstract art: the image has a certain prettiness, even beauty, and would not be out of place in a contemporary art gallery. In reality, it's a microscopic section from the biopsy, and the geographic features are created by the clumps, ribbons, and whorls of disorganized, pushing cancer cells.

Dr. Canning clears her throat and picks up her laser pointer, which she uses to point out the features of this undiscovered world.

"Here we see severe nuclear atypia ... over here, increased mitoses ..."

The red laser dot settles on an area where there is a dark island in the middle of a river.

"And here, a beautiful example of intravascular invasion." It's a clump of cancer cells plugging a blood vessel. She beams, like a tour guide proudly showing off a landmark.

She turns off the pointer and stares at us.

"In summary, it's a poorly differentiated squamous cell carcinoma."

A *squame* again. They're everywhere in the body: Betty, with her *squame* coiled inside her beret, and Matthew, with his lung lizard.

The patient definitely has cancer. Death gives a thumbs-up sign.

"Any evidence of deep invasion?" asks Dr. Little.

"Fortunately, no."

That's a relief. Deep invasion into the distensible inner tubes of the penis, the tubes engorged to produce erection, would be a bad thing, as it would give the cancer access to a rich blood supply and make the risk of spread very high.

"Thanks," says Dr. Little, and, her testimony complete, Dr. Canning returns to her seat. I glance at her. How do pathologists cope with their power of rendering life-and-death judgments on patients they never meet in person – except in the mortuary? Does she sit by the fire at night, knitting her cares into endless ribbons of woolly scarf? Or does she toss back thimbleful after thimbleful of sherry?

"Dr. Raj, can we look at the imaging?"

Dr. Raj, the radiologist, is the next witness. He quickly licks pizza juice off his fingers, goes to the podium, and presses a button. The pink blob dissolves. In its place is a stark greyscale image showing globules of varying shades of grey floating in an outer casing. It's a slice through the patient's CT scan: the casing is the skin, the globules his internal organs.

Dr. Raj scrolls through slices, using the red laser to identify organs while making brief comments about their health.

"Kidneys appear normal, as do adrenals ... aorta slightly distended but within normal limits ... incidental finding of granuloma in spleen ... here we can follow the ureters ..."

As he scrolls through the slices, the organs come to stuttering animated life, like images in those early movies created by rotating cards in a carnival peepshow. The kidneys and liver swell and contract, the bowel twists and swirls, and the aorta pulses.

Here is the reductionism of modern medicine carried to its extreme. There's no sense that these images, or the specimen shown earlier by the pathologist, have any connection to a human being. There's no face, no name, no personality. Patients' bodies are reduced to pathological and anatomic data – the epitome of the "case." Here, behind the doors of the conference room, the notion that patients are human beings who might want to have a say in their treatment is a foreign concept. On the rare occasion when patients make an appearance, it's not for them to be asked what they would like done, but simply to be checked for a pathological finding. At a breast conference I attended, women were shuffled into a side room outside the main conference room where, after the details of their cases were presented, a parade of doctors saw them – not to meet a person but instead to check for a questionably enlarged lymph node or lump in the breast. Sometimes the doctors engaged in a game of "find the lump," smiling in self-satisfied triumph when they discovered it and flashing frowns of barely concealed scorn at those who couldn't. I remember the anxious, cowed look on the faces of these women who had become living pathological specimens.

Occasionally there's a hint of a person connected to the data. Like today: Dr. Raj's pointer lingers on the liver, where he points out some streaks of fat, a common finding in heavy alcohol users.

"Oh yeah," says Dr. Little, "forgot to mention this guy's a boozer. Lives in a trailer."

A barely suppressed titter travels through the room. One of the most distasteful aspects of these conferences is the ease with which details of patients' private lives become fodder for humour – especially when those lives are remote from the comfortable, privileged stratum occupied by the specialists in the room, nowhere better represented than in the doctors' parking garage, with its array of gleaming high-end automobiles. Less fortunate guys who live boozy lives in trailer parks are beneath us. Or are they? Alcoholism and substance abuse are rampant in medicine.

There's also the suggestion that the patient is to blame for his cancer, stemming from the long-held belief that penile cancer is associated with the poor hygiene expected of someone who lives in a trailer. As long ago as the 1930s, public health officials, building on the associations between unsanitary living conditions and infectious diseases, conjectured that cancer was cultivated by uncleanliness and bad habits. In the case of smoking, such conjectures proved correct, but such attitudes led to the widespread "you brought it on yourself" mentality that still pervades attitudes to cancer and causes needless and undeserved guilt and shame among patients.

Dr. Raj points out the penis, a silvery discarded condom, reposing on the scrotum. A fuzzy black spider grips one side.

"Here's the cancer," he says. "Confined to the penis. There's no evidence for metastases."

His testimony complete, Dr. Raj goes to the side table and selects another slice of pizza.

One of the medical oncologists, a smart-ass fond of challenging the pathologists and radiologists, pipes up in a whiny, nasal voice.

"Hold on, didn't I see an enlarged lymph node?"

Dr. Raj returns to the podium.

"Where?"

"Over there, the lower pelvis."

Pizza in one hand, Dr. Raj scrolls through the images again.

"No, I think it's just a blood vessel."

"Funny place for a blood vessel."

Dr. Raj shrugs and resumes his seat.

Dr. Little resumes the podium. "To summarize, it looks like this fellow's got a T1N0M0 penile cancer."

His eyes scan the room and fix on a lean, gangly young man with an unruly crop of black hair and oversized round glasses. He's the junior trainee in urology.

"Dr. Tan, do you think this patient's curable?"

"T1. No spread. Sure," says Dr. Tan.

"Good lad." Dr. Little nods.

At the confirmation of cure, Death throws up his hands in a disappointed manner and disappears.

"So how would you cure him?"

Dr. Tan presses his lips together and scratches his cheek.

"Dr. Tan?"

There's silence as all eyes focus on young Dr. Tan. He shifts in his seat. His Adam's apple quivers like a turkey's wattle. The pungent aroma of stale cheese sits heavily in the air.

His discomfort instantly triggers a memory from my summer studentship in the cancer clinic. On my very first day, a sunny June morning, I sat in the back row of a similarly dark conference room at the Gynecological Tumour Board. The screen depicted another pink continent – on that occasion, a biopsy of a cervix cancer – and suddenly the professor of gynecology, a short bald man with a long neck, swivelled in his seat in the front row, fixed his ostrich eyes on me, and asked me what I would do. As all eyes in the room skewered me; my heart pounded, and sweat sprouted onto my palms.

I knew nothing about cervix cancer. Of course, he must have known this. I detected a sadistic glint in his eyes. He was playing with me, enjoying the sight of me squirm. After a moment of silence, the ostrich snorted, smirked, and fixed his gaze on another victim.

It was the first of countless public interrogations in conference rooms and hospital corridors.

Doctor, what would you do?

Doctor, tell me how would you handle this?

Doctor, are you sure about that?

Doctor, your patient just died!

This style of questioning is ingrained in medical training. It's a lefto-ver from days when medical services, often headed by ex-World War II servicemen like McCutcheon, were run like the military, and medical professors behaved like Marine sergeants drilling their recruits. For me, it evokes unpleasant memories of the boys' school I attended in England, run on similar principles of humiliation and punishment. There, an in-nocent misstep could land you a sarcastic taunt or a flick of the cane from the masters. The goal was to "make a man of you." In medicine, it's supposed to help you think on your feet, prepare for situations in which there's no time for drawn-out consideration, when a life hangs in the balance. Very often though, it's simply a sadistic game in which the questioner re-enacts his or her own youthful torments.

My own experiences with sarcastic humiliation, both at school and in medical training, have left me with a reflex dread of being called on which has lasted to this day. Over the years I've developed some strategies for coping, the most useful of which is to avoid the temptation to pre-varicate or hedge and to answer with an honest "I don't know" or "I'm not sure." An admission of ignorance is usually enough to quieten the interrogator.

Today it's poor Dr. Tan's turn.

"Ah ... excision?" he croaks.

Dr. Tan hasn't yet mastered another strategy: temporize by repeating the details of the case out loud while mentally formulating a response.

Dr. Little's face twists into a look of disdain, even disgust.

"Ex-cision??" he says with melodramatic sarcasm. An excision is a minor procedure that would remove just the tumour but maybe not all the cancer.

"Oh – then I guess a resection?"

"Guess?? You *guess* about cancer treatment?"

Dr. Tan twitches and slithers lower in his seat. He's regressed to a panicked schoolboy.

"Can anyone help Dr. Tan?"

The senior resident, a burly man with a chin of unshaven stubble and a nervous tic of scratching his hairy forearms, speaks up.

"The standard of care for penile cancer is penectomy," he intones in a flat voice, as though reciting a scriptural passage.

"Good. Dr. Tan, better bone up on the penis."

A quiet titter travels through the room. Unaware of his joke, Dr. Little looks momentarily startled.

"I'll book this fellow for a radical. Any objections?"

His eyes rapidly sweep round the room.

"Great."

He slams the file shut with the authority of a judge concluding a trial. Case closed.

"Next case?"

Hold on. Shouldn't there be more discussion of this case? Radiation will cure a penile cancer of this size, and cure it without the drastic step of removing the penis. During my career, I've treated several cases with success.

As the itchy senior resident recites the details of the next case, frustration rises inside me. Why isn't this unfortunate man who lives in a trailer being given more options? What will be the impact of surgery? Life without a penis? How will he pee? Have sex? Why, as happens so often in these conferences, are we being asked to merely rubber-stamp Dr. Little's opinion? My anger is intensified by Dr. Little's abruptness, which, as on many previous occasions, doesn't invite discussion.

Should I speak up? That old timidity born of previous humiliations grips me in its paralysing embrace. Maybe one of my colleagues will respond. I glance sideways at my fellow radiation oncologists, who must also know that radiotherapy is an option. One of them is flicking through Facebook posts on his phone; the other, belly full of pizza, is nodding off.

The resident continues to drone the details of his case.

Finally, I can't stand it any longer. I raise my hand. As I do so, a sticky film of sweat peels in my armpit.

Dr. Little swivels his eyes on me.

"Yes?"

"Can we go back to that last case for a minute. He might be a good candidate for radiation."

Dr. Little looks stunned.

"Radiation?" he says, like it's leprosy. "What would that do for him?"

"I've had several cases that were cured."

"*Cure?*" he says.

"Sure."

"Have you any evidence for that?"

"There's a series of cases from Manchester ..."

"*Manchester?*" Dr. Little's tone makes it sound like a primitive village in some remote outback. He's unaware, or pretending to be unaware, that Manchester's long-established Christie Hospital and Holt Radium Institute is one of the world's leading cancer research centres. Several of my radiation oncology mentors trained there.

"Come on. You can't extrapolate from *Manchester*," he says, implying Mancunians have a different species of penis from North Americans.

"Their data shows that radiation cures a high proportion of cases like this."

"Ah. But not all."

I muster a polite smile.

"With all due respect, surgery doesn't cure everyone either." A disgruntled murmur runs through the surgeons, like I've uttered heresy.

I've seen several unfortunate men whose cancers returned after penectomy. They came to me for palliative radiation for painful, stinking,
bleeding growths sprouting from the stump of the penis.

"It gives him a better chance."

"I'm not sure about that."

Dr. Little and I exchange hostile glares.

Our interchange reflects the old, deep-seated conflict between
operative and non-operative treatments for cancer that emerged soon
after the discovery of radiotherapy. The advantage of radiotherapy in
curing cancer without the use of mutilating surgery was recognized at
the beginning of the twentieth century and led some surgeons to adopt
radiation enthusiastically. At one European hospital, a surgeon chortled, "We no longer operate; we radiate!" For a time, surgeons acquired
radium and performed their own radiotherapy. Later, a new, separate
breed of medical specialists, radiotherapists (later called radiation oncologists), emerged, and threatened surgeons' supreme position in the
cancer universe. The threat came not just from radiation's claims to cure
cancer without cutting: it was also economic, as radiation robbed surgeons of lucrative operations. By the late twentieth century, surgeons
and radiotherapists had formed into two camps reflected in today's seat-
ing alignment at the conference.

Of course, surgery and radiotherapy are not always antagonists. Most
surgeons accept that radiation has a special role in treating cancers in
a body site where surgery would result in significant loss of function:
for example, for cancer of the larynx, where radiotherapy preserves the
voice, and for anal cancer, where it preserves the normal bowel passage.
Radiation oncologists acknowledge removal is better for large cancers,
where the chance of cure with radiation is low. In between, there are
a whole slew of cancers, such as those on the penis, where controversy
continues, partly because of conflicting evidence in each specialty's literature. Surgical journals are biased towards research favouring surgery, just
as radiation journals favour radiotherapy. In a phenomenon common to
all modern medical specialties, surgeons and Rad Oncs tend to hunker

in their own silos and read only their own journals, which are biased towards their approaches.

Controversies such as the question of the best treatment for penile cancer could be resolved by a randomized trial, in which patients with identical stages of cancer are randomly allocated to radiation or surgery. A randomized trial would provide the definitive, gold-standard answer of the treatments' equivalence or difference. There's never been a randomized trial of radiation and surgery for penile cancer, partly because the relative rarity of the cancer makes recruitment of patients difficult, and partly because of the reluctance of both surgeons and radiation oncologists to submit patients to random allocation for a treatment they don't like. It takes superhuman will power and good faith to submit a patient to a treatment with which one doesn't agree.

I turn to my radiation oncology colleagues for support. The drowsy one has stirred, but is staring hard at the floor. The other notices my glance and looks up from his phone.

"I don't know. Radiation to the penis is technically challenging," he says.

I resist the urge to kick him.

He's right though. For radiation, the penis must be immobilized in a rigid plastic cylinder that holds it away from the body. Coaxing a flaccid penis into the cylinder and keeping it there for the duration of treatment is often difficult. But it's not impossible.

"That doesn't mean we shouldn't give it a try," I say.

"Personally, I wouldn't waste the time," he says, his eyes dropping back to the screen.

Would he say the same if the cancer was on his penis? Or his father's?

My colleague's lack of support revs my engines.

"If radiation doesn't cure the cancer, he can have salvage surgery later," I continue.

The word "salvage" animates the surgeons, who stare at me with looks of frank hostility. They don't like to have surgery spoken of as a clean-up modality.

"By then, it's too late. The cancer will have spread," says the senior resident.

"Not always. The Manchester data shows that if the patients are monitored carefully, and the penis is removed at the first sign of recurrence, the survival will be the same as the patients who had the penis removed at the beginning."

At another mention of "Manchester," Dr. Little's eyeballs rotate first skyward, eliciting a titter from his colleagues, and then swivel down to fix on me.

"I'm not having this man get his penis fried."

The word "fried" triggers me as much as "salvage" inflames the surgeons. I hate the use of thermal imagery for radiation side effects. It just serves to scare patients and diminishes our modality to some kind of primitive medical barbeque. Naturally, there will be side effects, such as pain with urination, and redness, possibly blistering, of the skin, but these will dissipate a few weeks after treatment.

"He'll get some temporary side effects, sure. And the data shows the risk of long-term side effects is less than 5 per cent."

"Doesn't seem like 5 per cent around here. Maybe you fellows should get your radiation equipment checked."

Loud guffaws of laughter erupt from the surgeons.

"Look, we got six other cases to discuss," says Dr. Little. "This guy's booked for surgery."

"Won't surgery have side effects too?"

"Like what?"

"Like the impact on sexual functioning."

At the s-word, the room falls silent. Dr. Canning draws her cardigan closer. Despite the topic of these rounds being cancers of the genitourinary tract, sex is rarely, if ever, discussed.

"Sex? Come on. This guy lives in a *trailer*."

Louder guffaws from the surgeons.

"Settle down, settle down." Dr. Little is now the speaker of an unruly parliament.

Suddenly Dr. Wong, a petite woman sitting aside in one corner, raises her hand. "Excuse me, but does anyone know what the patient wants?"

The hubbub stops. All eyes turn to Dr. Wong like she's made a revolutionary utterance.

"I haven't discussed my plan with him yet," says Dr. Little.

"Well, is there any harm in sending the patient to Dr. Hayter just for a consultation and then letting him make up his own mind?"

She's hit on a brilliant way out of the impasse. The tension dissipates into nods and grunts of agreement, even from some of the surgeons.

Sensing sedition in his own ranks, Dr. Little raises his hands in mock surrender.

"Okay, okay. I'll send the guy to you for a consultation. His surgery won't be done for a week or so anyway. Now let's move on."

As the resident continues his description of the next case, I scrawl the patient's name and ID number on a wedge of paper plate.

A week later, the patient still hasn't got an appointment to see me. I ask Ivy to look him up in the computer and find out what's happened.

Ivy locates the information. She turns to me with a sheepish smile.

"Looks like Dr. Little performed surgery two days ago."

A couple of weeks later, I spot Dr. Little seated in the hospital cafeteria, head down over a bowl of spaghetti, shovelling forkfuls of noodles into his mouth. The sight of him reawakens the anger I felt when I learned the patient had his penis lopped off without a radiation consultation.

I pause by the cafeteria door, wondering if I should confront him. Like my colleagues, I normally let skirmishes with surgeons slide by without comment. Speaking up risks further humiliation or even ostracism. Surgeons, after all, are the source of our patients and thus our livelihood.

But there's something about this incident that's different. It's not only his dismissive attitude in conference, but also the blatant lie of agreeing to a radiation consultation followed by the colossal hubris of removing a man's penis without giving him options.

There are other men with penile cancer. I don't want it to happen to them. I also don't want him to think we Rad Oncs are pushovers.

My actor's training kicks in. I take a big breath, stand up tall, stride over, and slide onto the seat opposite him.

"Hi."

He looks up with a scowl.

"What's up?" he says, wiping tomato sauce from his chin with a paper napkin.

"Just wondering what happened with that case of penis cancer we discussed a couple of weeks ago at rounds?"

"Which case?"

"The guy who lives in a trailer."

"Oh, that one," he says with a smirk. "What about him?"

"You were to send him to me for a radiation consult."

"Was I?"

"Yes. The conference agreed. He never came. You went ahead with the penectomy."

He wipes his mouth, tosses the napkin and cutlery into the plastic bowl, and folds it over. There's a loud crunching sound as he flattens it with his hand.

"Oh yeah," he smiles in mock innocence. "Golly, I don't know what happened. I asked my secretary to set up an appointment with you. Must have fallen through the cracks."

I might have expected this response. Blaming secretarial lapses is a time-honoured way for doctors to pass the buck.

He stands up. "I'll speak to Melody about it. Have a great day."

He turns, performs a slam dunk with the garbage into a can, and marches out of the cafeteria.

7

The Confused Patient

My fears about the urologist are confirmed when I discover he's started my father on a testosterone blocker alone. Cripes. Doesn't he know about the study showing total blockade gives a longer period of remission? I'm tempted again to call him, but memories of unpleasant skirmishes with surgeons restrain me. Instead, I adopt an approach often used by my mother, an approach that in hindsight seems ashamedly passive-aggressive: I go formal. I compose a letter on my office letterhead to my parents, as if I'm writing a letter to one of my own patients. I explain the procedure and benefits of total blockade.

A couple of weeks later my mother replies. She's mentioned total blockade to the doctor. All he said was "I'm aware of it." He doesn't change the treatment.

My dismay softens when she mentions that since starting the blocker, my father feels more energetic, and recent lab tests show his acid phosphatase level has fallen – an indication his disease is reacting. Under these circumstances, I decide not to stir things further. Total blockade can always be introduced later.

I decide to focus on the area where I have the greatest competence: radiation. His energy is improved, but his pain persists. As I'd suggested at Christmas, my father needs radiation to his spine.

Radiation has been recognized as a useful treatment for pain from bone metastases since the earliest days of radiotherapy. In 1903, Toronto

X-ray pioneer John McMaster wrote, "Opiates may be laid aside very soon after beginning X-ray treatment." His comment underscored an important additional benefit of radiation: the relief of pain allowed patients to wean off narcotic painkillers and their sedating side effects. In my own practice, I've often witnessed seemingly miraculous effects of radiation on pain that allow patients to discontinue painkillers entirely.

Despite its established usefulness, many doctors remain ignorant about the use of radiation for bone pain. I've given talks about palliative radiation to family doctors and noted looks of surprise, even scepticism, when I describe its role in relieving pain. They're stuck in an unfortunate mindset of thinking only drugs will help. Worse still, I've been summoned to the bedsides of many cancer patients dying in wracking pain that is unresponsive to painkillers. Their pain could have been relieved months earlier if a radiation oncologist had been consulted.

I hope my father's urologist doesn't share this ignorance. I want my father to see a radiation oncologist to help his pain.

There's another factor at play. Besides my doctor's reasoning, the son in me wants affirmation of his chosen career. My father's reaction to my career choice was lukewarm at best. Now's the chance for him to see my specialty up close, to recognize its value, to maybe even be impressed by its methods and results.

I call my mother and suggest a radiation consultation.

"Yes, Daddy saw the radiation doctor yesterday. A Dr. Keith."

Relief sweeps over me. The radiation oncology community in Canada is small. I've met Dr. Keith at conferences. He's a short, stocky Brit who struck me as a kind, sensitive man cut from the same cloth as Dr. Friar, the radiation oncologist whom I saw stroking the patient's hand during my summer internship.

My gladness dissipates when my mother tells me he's booked my father for ten treatments. Ten? I almost drop the receiver.

During my residency, ten daily treatments for patients with bone pain was standard, yet something about it bothered me and many other Rad Oncs. It didn't seem right to haul patients in pain in day after day, subjecting them to the added discomfort of bumpy car rides and transfers onto treatment couches. Many of them had advanced cancer with multiple bone metastases, and by the time they finished radiation to one area, another area started to cause pain, necessitating another two-week round of trips. In 1986, when I was midway through my residency, Dr. Pam Price and colleagues at the Royal Marsden Hospital in London published a landmark study in which patients with cancerous bone pain were randomly allocated to either a single radiation treatment or one treatment each day for ten days. The study showed a single treatment was just as effective as ten in relieving pain. To produce equivalent pain relief, the single dose was stronger than a normal daily dose but did not seem to produce additional side effects. I spent several months at the Marsden when I completed training in Canada, so I was very familiar with these results and their potential impact on the quality of life of patients, who were saved from making multiple uncomfortable trips to the radiation department. When I returned to Canada I adopted it as my standard approach, as many of my Canadian colleagues had already done.

Dr. Keith's plan doesn't completely surprise me. Many of my radiation colleagues are very conservative and slow to adopt new techniques, from a combination of scepticism of new research and comfort with regimes they've used for years that give predictable results. On one hand, their conservatism is admirable: radiation is a powerful, potentially destructive tool that should only be applied with caution. On the other, it sometimes blinds them to the possibility of improving the quality of their patients' lives. The doctor's own comfort with a safe approach takes precedence over improvements in patient comfort. They prefer the tried but not necessarily true. In the case of radiation for bone metastases, in the late 1980s a new truth about radiation for bone pain was emerging. The efficacy of single treatments has since been confirmed in many studies.

My father's pain is severe. I don't want him going for uncomfortable car rides every day for a week when there's a simpler, equally effective alternative.

I've come face to face with a decades-old conflict in the radiation oncology world.

~

It's Thursday morning, and my busy review clinic has been brought to
a stuttering, screeching halt by a patient who won't leave until she gets
"answers."

Review clinic is a regular event on a Rad Onc's weekly calendar. Apart
from palliative treatments, a course of radiation typically takes several
weeks, and every patient is seen once weekly by his or her doctor to review
progress and to help with side effects – both physical and emotional. The
physical side effects of radiation are bad enough, but in review the doctors and nurses have to also deal with psychic wounds in patients still
raw from the recent diagnosis of cancer. Little wonder that in the forge
of a course of radiation, patients form strong bonds with their doctors,
nurses, and radiation therapists. As patients' mettle is tested, revealing
hidden strengths or weaknesses, it becomes impossible to regard them as
mere "cases" any more – just as they start to see their doctors and therapists as more than anonymous white coats. In my experience, the bonds
that form between radiation oncologists and their patients can be very
strong and lasting. Radiation may have a very technical public brand, but
the review clinic shows its human side.

Review is also the closest the radiation department comes to an emergency department. It's held in a dark rabbit warren of rooms across the
hall from the radiation machines and provides rapid access to a doctor
for patients with unexpected problems. On a busy day, it's crammed with
patients both waiting for their regular weekly review and requiring urgent attention. The urgent cases, with problems such as nausea, pain,
bleeding, or diarrhoea, sit in wheelchairs or lie on stretchers in curtained
alcoves. It's often filled with a sad chorus of humans in distress: moans,
retching, coughing. Because of its dark, crowded, chaotic environment,

the review clinic at one former hospital where I worked earned the nick-name "the pit." Unless it was their duty day, nurses and doctors alike avoided "the pit."

The radiation nurse – a nurse with special training in radiation side effects – is the ringleader of this spectacle. It's her – and it usually is a her – job to put the patients in the examining rooms, perform an as-sessment, give me a short briefing, and provide support. When I was a fledgling oncologist, such nurses were fonts of wisdom and common sense from whom I learned a great deal. They often knew secret lore for dealing with side effects and helpful tactics for dealing with emotional issues. Their job is to keep the clinic moving along by making sure all the rooms remain filled with patients – and by making sure I don't linger too long with any one patient.

But today I have to linger. My patient Tasmeen, a forty-five-year-old high school chemistry teacher who's getting radiation to the left breast af-ter removal of a small cancer, has accused me of withholding information from her. She's usually open and friendly, but today there's a tightness to her face and body that betray an inner agitation.

"How come you didn't tell me?"

"Tell you what?"

"My cancer is so bad."

I quickly review her file. Just as I thought: T1N0M0 well-differentiated infiltrating ductal carcinoma of the left breast, removed with clear mar-gins, getting routine post-operative radiotherapy to the breast to prevent recurrence.

"You have stage one breast cancer. The prognosis is very good."

"Then how come you're giving me so many treatments?"

"Uh ... you're getting the standard number of treatments we use for breast cancer."

"No, I'm not. I was chatting to the woman sitting next to me in the waiting room. She's got breast cancer too, but she's getting only sixteen treatments. Why am I getting twenty-five? What are you hiding from me? Is my cancer worse than you said? Am I going to die?"

She stares at me over the top of her half-moon glasses like she would at one of her pupils. Her normally soft brown eyes constrict to black dots.

Uh-oh. Tasmeen has a bad case of waiting-room syndrome.

Doctors tend to ignore the power of the waiting room. They stride through it as if it's some Beckett-esque no-man's-land where patients just sit in numbed silence and wait, wait, and wait some more. But sometimes I've lingered on its edges and observed it's quite the opposite – a meeting place, an agora, teeming with human drama.

Over there, a young man cradles an older woman – his mother? – in his arms. She weeps, perhaps reeling from an assault of bad news. Behind them, another tableau of sorrow: three women huddle around a thin, bearded elderly man. I glimpse his pale, anxious face between their shoulders. Nearby, two white-haired ladies chat amiably as they knit furiously from balls of wool unravelling in their laps. One of them spots me and waves her knitting needle. I recognize her as one of my patients, and I smile and return the wave. She turns to her friend and whispers something. Their bellies heave with giggles. Are they gossiping about me?

Closer to me, two men with dark bushy moustaches gab and gesticulate in a manner reminiscent of a comedy duo from a 1930s film. They're perhaps debating politics or sports. In the aisle, a middle-aged man in a dark suit and slicked-back hair stomps up and down, looking impatiently at his watch and shooting angry looks at the receptionist, who keeps her gaze fixed on her computer screen.

In between the family groups, I spot solitary, lonely figures, some absent-mindedly flipping through the tattered pages of old magazines, others simply staring blankly at a TV screen suspended in one corner of the ceiling. It shows endless loops of infomercials extolling the wonders of the hospital's various services. Most of the time it's filled with the smiling face of the hospital's CEO, mouthing words that, above the hubbub of the waiting room, nobody can hear. I've never seen anybody paying serious interest to it, and I've often silently stewed over the money spent on propaganda that could have been used to directly help patients. It's a surreal import from a third-world dictatorship.

A young man in an apron with red pinstripes – probably a med-school wannabe – weaves a cart laden with a coffee urn and a plate of cookies up and down the aisles, offering treats and grins. And over there, yes, that's the solitary, shrouded figure of Death, sizing up the occupants of the waiting room.

Doctors ignore this hive of human activity, but fictional representations of cancer treatment often emphasize the meaningful connections of the waiting room. One of the few plays to depict radiation therapy, Adam Pettle's *Therac-25*, which has received several successful international productions, charts the course of a friendship and tentative romance between two strangers, Alan and Moira, in the waiting room at Princess Margaret Hospital in Toronto. Alan jokes he likes to keep the radiation machine – "that monster that treats me" – waiting. They make secretive jokes about the other patients, calling one "the mantis" because she prays out loud before her treatment.

The Doctor, a 1991 film starring William Hurt, depicts the Scrooge-like transformation of Dr. Jack McKee from a blunt, arrogant, apparently heartless surgeon to a caring, compassionate, joyful human through his personal experience with laryngeal cancer. During Jack's radiation treatment, more screen time is devoted to the waiting room than the treatment bunker. Jack's experience of the suffering of his fellow patients, and his friendship with June, a young woman with a brain tumour, become important catalysts for his personality change.

Radiotherapy is administered over several weeks, and patients encounter each other daily, so it's not uncommon for real friendships to develop. I've witnessed pairs of patients, previous strangers, exchange contact information at the end of their treatments, much as new friends might do on disembarking a cruise ship.

Such friendships can be extremely helpful in easing the passage through radiation. One patient who's a week ahead of another patient can reassure the other that the looming side effects are not as bad as she fears.

But waiting-room chats can also be unhelpful, such as the one this morning. Tasmeen has compared notes with another patient, and her discovery that she's getting a prolonged treatment has aroused both fear and mistrust.

Sometimes encounters in review can be so brief that I can remain standing. A quick check to be sure the patient is okay, and I'm off to see the next patient.

Tasmeen's insistent look tells me I need to spend more time with her. I roll a stool and sit in front of her.

"Uh, well, there's different ways of giving radiation."

It's a sop, but in the hurried atmosphere of the review clinic, with patients waiting, there's always a temptation to abbreviate and simplify explanations.

She's not going to let me off so easily

"She has exactly the same cancer as me. Why am I getting two weeks' more treatment? Please just tell me the truth, doctor."

Tasmeen has a very common concern, one that cuts across medical specialties and arises any time patients witness doctors giving different treatments to patients with the same disease. To answer her question, it's necessary to reach back to the early history of radiotherapy. Very soon after the discovery of X-rays in 1895 and radium in 1898, doctors recognized their therapeutic potential. Because radiation caused harm to healthy tissues, one of the key challenges was how to deliver a curative dose to the cancer while limiting collateral damage. The delicate balance between cure and toxicity remains at the heart of radiation practice and research today. One of the strategies to assure safety is to give radiation over time, rather than in a single dose, using small daily amounts that build up to a cumulative total dose.

A famous experiment confirming this approach used unfortunate French rams submitted to sterilization using radiation. If experimenters zapped their scrotums with a single blast, the reproductive cells died, but at the cost of a nasty blistering burn. The poor rams wandered around for days with inflamed scrotums chafing between their hind legs. Yet if the scientists spread the treatment out over a few days, radiation had the desired effect of sterilization but without blistering of the scrotum. The rapidly dividing reproductive cells were a surrogate for cancer cells; those of the skin, for healthy tissue. From this experiment, and similar observations in humans undergoing cancer treatment, the concept of "fractionation" – or splitting the total radiation dose into small daily doses (fractions) – became accepted practice for patients receiving potentially curative radiotherapy. Every radiotherapy waiting room should really display an icon of these heroic rams who sacrificed their gonads for the sake of human health.

While radiation doctors agreed on the basic concept, they did not agree on the specifics: the best overall duration of a course of radiation and the exact number of fractions into which a total dose should be divided. By the late twentieth century, the practice of radiotherapy evolved into two main schools: one based in the US, which advocated giving radiotherapy over a long six- or seven-week period using moderate doses per fraction; and the other, based in Europe, favouring shorter, three- to five-week courses using higher daily doses.

It's the late 1980s, and I'm a final-year trainee in radiation oncology, with enough experience to write radiation prescriptions on my own, though they still need to be signed off by a senior staff doctor.

It's early evening, and I sit alone at a desk in the radiation workroom, a windowless space lit with fluorescent strips deep in a maze of corridors behind the radiation treatment units. A constant faint hum surrounds me – the sound of electrical power surging through cables, accelerating electrons towards targets in the heads of the treatment units, where their impact generates cancer-destroying beams of photons. Cut off from any external landmarks, I feel like I'm on the lower deck of a ship, hearing only the low drone of turbines.

Charts printed with rows and columns of radiation data stare down at me from the walls like inscriptions in an ancient temple. Indeed, this workroom is the inner sanctum of radiotherapy, where measurements, doses, plans, and calculations coalesce to the final radiation prescription handed to the radiation technologists performing the rites of treatment.

A blank radiation prescription form sits on the desk in front of me. The patient is a sixty-two-year-old man with a cancer of the bladder. He's refused removal of the bladder and is to receive curative radiotherapy appropriate for his stage of cancer. I'm trying to decide what radiation dose to prescribe. Should I do as one of my European-trained mentors suggests, and give him twenty treatments, or should I follow the advice of a teacher who studied in the US and give him thirty? Each claims his treatment works as well as the other, with similar side effects. I've read the papers supporting their respective positions. There's data to support both approaches, but none is from large clinical trials where patients are allocated randomly to twenty or thirty treatments. The existing data comes from "single-arm" studies at individual hospitals that summarize the results for a group of patients treated in a similar way. Doctors at different hospitals claim their results are better or at least equivalent to those of another hospital, but their conclusions are tainted by bias of the characteristics of the patients in their institution.

As I try to decide what to prescribe, I tap my pen in a staccato telegraph on the counter. Fatigue from a long day seeing patients blunts my thinking. I'm anxious about my upcoming exams in radiation oncology. What will I say if I'm presented with a case of bladder cancer like this? With good reason, examiners do not like an indecisive candidate. Will my examiner be a former Brit who favours four-week treatment or a Yank who thinks anything less than six weeks is useless?

Maybe if I rest for a minute my mind will clear. I lay my arms on the table, rest my head, and close my eyes. The electrical hum around me surges.

I'm stretched out on a wooden recliner on the deck of a ship somewhere in a vast, grey ocean. As the ship heaves, the horizon bobs and twists in the distance. I notice life rings stamped with *SS RADIATION* hung on the railing.

A short, wiry, red-headed man wearing a bright tartan kilt swaying under a white coat strolls up to me.

"Acch, me lad, buck up!" he says. "There's nothing wrong with a short, sharp course of treatment."

He makes a rapid chopping gesture with his hands.

"Get it over with as fast as possible."

His sharp consonants stir the figure lounging on the chair next to me: a tall, lean fellow wearing a crumpled linen suit. "Don't listen to Shorty," he drawls, pushing his Panama hat back, revealing a long face with a droopy white moustache.

He fans himself with a blank radiation prescription sheet.

"Jus' thinkin' about what he says makes me hot. You're in charge of a radiation machine, not a barbeque."

Shorty stamps his foot.

"Cancer's a vile thing. It needs heat."

"Lookee. This young fellow knows his basics. If you shorten the treatment you have to increase the daily dose. And as everyone knows, the higher the daily dose, the greater the risk of side effects. Eh, son?"

I nod in agreement.

"And as Dr. Long should also know, if you keep the radiation area small, the risk of side effects is low," Shorty squeaks. "Keep your target volume as small as possible, lad, and you'll stay out of trouble."

Dr. Long fans himself more vigorously. "I've seen some of these tiny radiation fields. Dinky!" He stretches his arms wide. "You wanna cure cancer, you got to go big. Big!"

A young woman in a bikini with an American flag draped over her shoulders wanders across the deck and waves at us.

"You can't risk a Geographic Miss! But yeah, one thing's for sure, you go big, you got to keep your daily dose low."

Dr. Short wags a stubby finger. "So low you don't cure the cancer!"

"Stealth! You got to creep up on it unawares, hit it before it knows it's being hit. Bah! Shorty here thinks we're still in the war."

"What's the war got to do with it?" I ask.

"With bombs flyin' this way and that, those Brits needed to get their patients in and out of hospital as quick as possible."

Dr. Short twists in a sardonic bow.

"With all due respect to my American colleague, we were using short treatments well before the war."

"Figures. You Scots are as tight with your radiation as you are with your money."

Dr. Short twirls and almost levitates.

"Money? Glad you brought that up. Why don't you tell this lad the real reason why you Yanks stretch your treatments out?"

"What would that be?"

"Don't act coy. Don't you get paid for every visit? The more visits, the fatter your bank account. Isn't that so? Beware of greed, laddie. Where I work we get paid a salary, so the length of treatment has no effect on my income."

Dr. Long tilts a cocktail glass towards Dr. Short.

"Nothin' wrong with being paid handsomely for curing cancer."

Dr. Short pulls a flask from his sporran.

"Aaach. The time these poor lads and lassies with cancer have to spend away from their homes in your country is a crying shame," he says, taking a swig and wiping his lips. "Even in America, you don't have radiation machines on every corner. Every patient I've ever talked to prefers to come to the hospital for four weeks."

"Course they would," Dr. Long drawls, swirling his ice in his glass. "I've seen what passes for accommodation in Scotland. Drafty old hotels with cranky plumbing. No doubt the hospitals are the same. Down where I live, we treat our patients first class to fancy accommodations."

"For which they pay through their noses."

"Some consider it a vacation."

"Vacation? Cancer treatment?" Dr. Short snorts, then takes another swig.

"Forget about accommodation. The important thing is cure. Cure! Our results are just as good as yours."

"Now that's just plain horseshit."

Dr. Short coughs and sputters a spray of whisky. The two men glare at each other. They're going to come to blows.

"Look, you two, have you any idea how confusing this is to a trainee like me?" I say.

"No confusion in my mind," says Long, taking another sip.

"A little confusion's good for you, lad," says Short. "Helps you make up your mind for yourself. Makes a man of you."

He offers me the flask. I wave it away.

"It seems you guys have been fighting about this for decades. Why don't you do a proper study – a randomized trial? Half the patients get the short treatment, the other half the long. See if the cure rates are the same or not."

They stare at me as if I'm deranged.

"Did you say randomize?" says Dr. Long, like it's poison. "Randomize, and run the risk of half my patients getting fried to death?"

"And run the risk of not curing?" trills Dr. Short.

"It would settle the question once and for all. I don't know why you guys don't cooperate instead of bicker."

Dr. Long stands and leans over me. I smell liquor on his breath.

"My, my. I'd say you're getting a bit too big for your britches, son. Just do what I say. It'll keep you out of trouble."

With that, he stands up and lopes off unsteadily.

I stare at Dr. Short. A smile appears on his face.

"Sure you don't want a dram of whisky, laddie? It would help calm your nerves."

"No thanks."

I sit up and look at the horizon. "Where's this ship heading, anyway?" I say, gazing at the expanse of ocean.

"Canada. Your home. Like in most things, you're kind of stuck between the British and American way of doing things. Kind of like the War of 1812, eh? Come to think of it, Canada would be the perfect place for that randomized trial you spoke of."

I pick up the blank prescription form.

"That'll never happen," I say. "Even if it does, it'll take years. Until then, what am I going to do with patients like this? What am I going to say on my exam?"

"Answer's staring you in the face."

He points to the demographic information in the patient's file.

"This fellow lives a hundred kilometres from your clinic. Is it really necessary to put him through an extra two weeks of bouncy car rides – especially when his bladder gets sore from the radiation?"

He gives me a wink, then lurches off along the deck.

I open my eyes, pick up my pen, and prescribe twenty treatments for the patient.

Dr. Short is right about the situation in Canada, where for many decades radiotherapy practice was a battleground for dominance between British and American traditions. The differences in practice between radiation doctors perplexed trainees like me but did force us into a deeper questioning of the available literature. It also had one very positive side: Canada was fertile ground for clinical trials that might resolve some of the questions. From witnessing different practices among their colleagues up close, Canadian radiation oncologists were more open to testing clinical questions than their British and American colleagues, who tended to be more entrenched in their views.

It took a shove from external economic and political factors to get research started. In the 1980s, increasing rates of cancer put pressure on the capacity of radiotherapy centres, which have only a finite number of treatment machines and treatment slots. In addition, radiotherapy was finding widening applications – particularly for women like Tasmeen with early stage breast cancer. In the 1970s, Vera Peters showed lumpectomy (removal of the tumour) followed by radiation cured the same proportion of women as mastectomy and saved women from the physical mutilation and emotional distress of breast removal. Her findings were met by scepticism and even hostility from surgeons who clung to the idea that the only sure cure for breast cancer was mastectomy. It was only after results from a (male-run) randomized trial in the mid-1980s showed the equivalence of breast-conserving therapy and mastectomy that surgeons began to adopt lumpectomy as standard treatment for women with early small breast cancers. Without radiation after lumpectomy, the risk of cancer recurrence in the breast approached 30 per cent. As more and more women sought cure without disfigurement, the floodgates opened, machines became backlogged, and patient queues grew. In Ontario, home to the world's largest centralized radiotherapy system, there was public outcry when patients had to be sent away from their home towns and sometimes to the United States for timely treatment.

At that time in Canada, the standard approach for post-operative radiation for breast cancer was an American-inspired twenty-five treatments over five weeks. In Europe, women often received treatment in as little as three weeks – with apparently the same results. If women with early breast cancer could be treated in three instead of five weeks, it would free up two weeks of slots on the radiation units, allow more women to be treated, shorten queues, and stop patients from being shuffled off to Buffalo. But were shorter treatments really as effective and safe as longer ones? Although some doctors were willing to shorten their regimes, others remained sceptical. Many were particularly concerned about using the higher daily doses needed in the shorter regime, since higher doses might result in a type of scarring called "woody fibrosis," where the entire breast became as rigid and hard as an overbaked loaf stuck to the chest. Over the years I'd seen a few women with this unpleasant side effect.

However, there was agreement that the question needed to be settled conclusively. As a result, the Ontario Clinical Oncology Group, led by doctors from McMaster University, began a clinical trial in which women who had undergone lumpectomy were randomly assigned to receive breast radiation in sixteen or twenty-five treatments.

It's easy to underestimate the challenges the team of investigators faced. To produce statistically meaningful results, they needed to recruit more than a thousand women, which entailed the cooperation of multiple oncologists in many centres. I was one of the doctors who participated. I supported the trial, but recruiting patients was more stressful than I anticipated. It taught me that the day-to-day running of clinical trials is much more challenging than I thought. Explanations of the rationale and procedure of the trial added an extra layer of time and complexity to a consultation. Beyond this, I had to relinquish my control over a patient's treatment and allow it to be determined by a higher power: the randomization process. At times I felt my role reduced to that of an army recruiter sizing up potential recruits and selling them on the benefits of enlistment.

I could see how difficult it was for the women too. Their reactions ranged from outright hostility – "No way you're using me as a guinea pig!" – to confusion. Despite explanations by me and the clinical-trial nurses, and review of a three-page consent form, they often misunderstood what was being asked of them – not surprising, since the form was in dense, complicated language. Even after taking the form away and studying it at home, many retained the idea that randomization meant they could choose their own treatment. Some who liked the idea of short treatment were disappointed and even backed out when they discovered they'd been randomized to the five-week regime. Other women participated enthusiastically, many with genuine excitement to be part of something that was pushing the boundaries of medical knowledge.

As the trial continued and the number of patients grew, suspense mounted. Would cure rates be the same? Would the shorter regime scar more breasts? The tension bubbled over one day when one of my colleagues, a notorious disbeliever in short fractionation who'd refused to participate in the trial, stormed into the clinic and pronounced in jubilant tones he'd heard there were more recurrences in the group receiving short treatment. "This trial should be stopped at once!" he thundered.

Of course, the organizers of the trial would never allow such preliminary and statistically meaningless data to leak out, but his anxiety infected me and awoke a niggling doubt that the shorter regime might be inferior to the longer. The stakes were high: patients' lives and, if not their lives, their breasts, for if a woman developed a recurrence in the breast, she required mastectomy. I had to ignore the naysayers and suppress my doubts, and instead focus on the bigger scientific question that could be answered only by analysing the results from the entire group of women being studied. A few interim recurrences in the short treatment had no bearing on the ultimate outcome. What mattered was whether there were a similar number of recurrences after the long treatment.

It's a credit to the generosity of women and the cooperative spirit of oncologists that it took only three-and-a-half years to recruit the patients needed. Other similarly ambitious cancer trials have taken up to ten years to accrue patients and sometimes have been abandoned without being completed.

Relief swept over me and the radiation oncology community when the final results showed there was no difference in cancer recurrence rates between the two groups. What about toxicity? The steering team of the trial had anticipated the results might founder on the question of breast scarring, so they had built careful assessment of the cosmetic appearance of the breast post-radiation into the trial. The assessment included blinded evaluation of photographs of the breasts of the participants after radiation. The fear that the larger fraction size in the group receiving the short course might produce greater scarring proved to be unfounded: nobody could tell whether a breast had been exposed to sixteen or twenty-five treatments.

After the publication of the results of this trial, the sixteen-fraction treatment was adopted as standard approach for women with early breast cancer in most centres across Canada. Much-needed space on treatment units was freed up, the queues were shortened, and women got their cancer treatment over with more quickly.

This study was important in another way: it demonstrated the feasibility of conducting multi-hospital trials of radiation-dose regimes. It stimulated similar trials for men with early stage prostate cancer, another cancer whose burgeoning incidence placed pressure on the radiation system and where there was similar controversy about the duration of radiation. A trial led by Princess Margaret Hospital showed equivalence for cure and toxicity for men randomly allocated to twenty or thirty-nine treatments. The twenty-fraction regime became standard, and men are now also able to complete their treatment more quickly than before.

I describe the breast cancer trial to Tasmeen. At the conclusion of my explanation, she leans forward with an even more insistent stare.

"Now I'm even more confused, doctor. You say sixteen treatments gives the same results as twenty-five. So why am I still getting twenty-five? What are you not telling me?"

"You remember we did a special CT scan to prepare your treatment?"

Her eyes widen in alarm.

"It showed more cancer?"

"No. No cancer. You have an excellent prognosis. The CT showed you have large breasts."

She frowns.

I explain that in any part of the body, as the volume of tissue receiving radiation increases, so does the risk of side effects. When we measured the volume of Tasmeen's breasts with the CT scan, their volume exceeded the threshold for using the large daily dose on the sixteen-treatment regime. A large daily dose might expose her to an increased risk of long-term side effects. Until there's better data on the effect of high daily doses on large breasts, it's better to be cautious and stick to the five-week treatment.

In the busyness of day-to-day practice, it's easy to overlook informing patients about adjustments in their treatment that are routine to me but have a major impact on them. It's related to a residuum of the paternalistic attitudes inculcated in me as a student: the doctor knows best, and patients should just go along and accept changes without question. But I know better: being busy is just an excuse, and every patient deserves to learn directly from me the reasons for such a significant change as extending the treatment from three to five weeks. Tasmeen's situation is a reminder of my failure to live up to my own principles. As I think of my ineptitude and the distress it has caused her, blood rises to my cheeks.

I wheel my stool closer to her.

"I'm very sorry," I say. "I usually find time to explain this after the CT and before treatment starts. I'm sorry I missed that. I understand why it would make you anxious."

"My cancer's definitely not worse?"

"Absolutely not."

Her face relaxes, and her mouth curves into a smile. Then a flush appears on her cheeks, and her body heaves with giggles.

"What's wrong?" I say.

"Goodness, doctor. You're the first man who ever told me I have large breasts."

8

The Interfering Child I

As with the urologist, I'm tempted to call my father's radiation oncologist and nudge him towards a single treatment. My temptation is stronger because I've met Dr. Keith and know he's friendly and approachable.

I look up Dr. Keith's number, pick up the phone, start to dial, then stop. What am I doing? I'm not my father's doctor. Dr. Keith is perfectly competent, with decades more experience than me. The decision about radiation is between him and my father, and my father has the final say. I have to remember what Ivy said to me about Peter: "It's his life."

I replace the receiver. Is my anxiety about my father's condition fuelling a need to control? More than that, is my temptation to intervene a perverse manifestation of my imposter syndrome? Am I just trying to show off my medical knowledge, to prove myself, to measure up?

Besides, how would I feel if some young Rad Onc who considered himself a hotshot called me up and asked me to change my radiation prescription for his relative?

I don't want to turn into a species I know well: the Interfering Son..

~

One sunny Sunday in mid-May, I'm out for an early morning walk on a meandering riverside path. As I stride through the fresh spring air, my face tingling in response to the sunshine, I see green shoots unfurling everywhere around me, and I'm enveloped in a cheerful chorus of happy birdsong.

Suddenly a discordant screech intrudes on this anthem. It's an electronic chirp from the pager strapped on my belt, an electronic crow whose impertinent caw is always a portent of danger for someone, somewhere. I squeeze its throat to silence it and gaze at its dull grey eye, where a series of numerals directs me to call the emergency department.

There's a perception among other medical specialists that we radiation oncologists have cushy jobs. Many of them think we have no contact with patients at all – we're just technicians who press buttons and pull levers at the helm of radiation machines. Those who are better informed know we see patients in person but still think of us as idlers because most of our practice involves outpatients seen in nine-to-five clinics. One colleague, a surgeon, always hailed me at the coffee shop in the hospital lobby with a cheery jibe, "Oh, you decided to come to work today?" The misconceptions arise from doctors' lack of exposure to radiation oncology in medical schools as well as from a certain deeply rooted need in doctors to put other doctors down. Doctors set up an imaginary hierarchy within the work ethic of medicine, with each specialty vying for top spot as to who works the hardest. Within this hierarchy, the almost invisible specialty of radiation oncology is an easy mark. Not immune to this attitude, radiation oncologists can sometimes be heard putting their diagnostic radiology colleagues down for sitting on their bums in quiet offices, staring at radiological ghosts of patients all day long, while we are out there on our feet seeing real people in fraught situations.

I chose the specialty partly because, as a father of two young children, I anticipated that I could be home most evenings in a way my father hadn't. I discovered quickly there's plenty of work that can easily intrude on home life: reviewing patients' test results; contouring tumours and healthy structures on scans; checking and signing off radiation plans;

answering phone calls from patients, families, and colleagues; and doing consultations on the hospital wards on inpatients who are too sick or frail to come to the clinic. There's also time needed to keep up with reading in the field to stay abreast of new knowledge and to prepare for teaching. On certain nights and weekends, I had to carry a pager as part of a roster of radiation oncologists on call for emergencies. I considered myself lucky to be able to take the pager home, instead of bunking in the hospital like some of my colleagues in other fields, and even luckier when a night went by without it bleeping its urgent summons. When it does go off though, it's usually a call to a difficult situation. When cancer comes calling after hours, it doesn't come with a polite knock on the door: it's more like a wrecking ball smashing through the wall.

Like today. An hour after my pager chirps, I'm standing in the ER, face to face with a young man with curly black hair and large brown eyes set in round wire frames. He stares at me, brow furrowed, his mouth a dark oval of astonishment.

"My dad has *cancer*?"

It's the third time in five minutes he's asked me this question.

"It certainly looks that way."

"*Cancer*?" he repeats, looking towards his father, an elderly man wearing a turban, lying on a stretcher in a curtained alcove. He's so thin his body looks like a deflated mannequin beneath the bed sheets. "Are you sure?"

"The scans point towards it," I say.

"It can't be. My dad's never been sick."

I understand his surprise. Earlier that day, Mr. Singh, like me, had set out for a morning walk in the spring sunshine. A few metres from his house, he'd stumbled and fallen to the pavement. When he tried to get up, his legs were so weak he couldn't stand without clinging onto a fence. A neighbour spotted his difficulty and called an ambulance. At the hospital, an urgent MRI scan has shown deposits of cancer throughout his spine. Our walks have now converged in the emergency room.

"Can you show me this MRI?"

"Okay." I lead him towards a desk, turn on a computer, and locate Mr. Singh's scan.

"Here's his spine," I say, scrolling through the sagittal view, which bisects the body into right and left sides. On an MRI, the spine shows as a gently curving stack of silver blocks.

"These are his vertebrae. Here are the healthy ones. But several are diseased. You can see tumours here, and here, and here," I say, indicating places where the blocks look more like burnt-out charcoal briquettes: black, fuzzy, and cracked.

There's a faint putrid smell. I turn and see the figure of Death looking over our shoulders, peering at the MRI with an expression of glee.

The young man gulps. "Are you sure you have the right patient?"

"Yes. And here's where the big problem is."

I indicate an area where one briquette is completely crushed, extruding itself into the spinal canal, the channel carrying the spinal cord, the thick cable that carries nerve impulses from the brain to the body, through the vertebrae. Black shards of tumour encase the cord, squeezing it to half its normal diameter. And now, on this second review of the scan, I spot a second similar area, further down in the spine, where another diseased vertebra compresses the spinal cord.

"Before today, was your dad having any pain?" I ask.

"He's been using a rub lately for some soreness."

"These tumours are pressing on the spinal cord. This explains your father's weak legs."

"I still don't get it. Where did they come from?"

I scroll sideways through the images. An indistinct grey blob appears in the upper part of the left lung.

"This is likely the origin. A cancer in the lung. Is your dad a smoker?"

The young man's gaze drops.

"Uh, yeah. But how did it get from there to here?" He points at the images of the spine.

"Likely through the blood. That's how most cancers spread."

His eyes expand and his body teeters slightly backward.

"My God."

"Are you okay?" I say, gripping his arm.

He recovers his balance. "What needs to be done?"

"The priority is to give him some radiation to his spine to stop these tumours from growing and pressing further on the spinal cord. With any luck, we can catch this early enough before there's more damage."

"*Radiation?* But you're not even sure he has cancer?"

"There's really nothing else that gives this picture."

"I can't believe it. How can we find out for sure?"

"The only way is to do a biopsy – take a sample of one of the tumours. But the results will take days to come back. We can't wait that long. He needs something done today to relieve the pressure on his spinal cord or he might get paralysed."

Death smiles and slips into a curtained alcove. The young man moves to one side of the stretcher and grips his father's hand.

"Radiation? No. No. I don't want him going through that."

Mr. Singh has the most common radiation oncology emergency, spinal cord compression, when a cancerous tumour in the spine infiltrates the spinal canal and presses on the spinal cord. Most commonly, the tumour is a metastasis from a primary cancer elsewhere in the body.

The announcement that "a cord compression's coming" causes a ripple of anxiety through the radiation department and is a rallying cry for doctors, nurses, and radiation therapists alike. It's all hands on deck: the doctor assigned the case prepares to do a quick assessment, the nurse arms himself with painkillers and steroids, the dosimetrists suspend their work on other patients, and the therapists clear an appointment on the treatment machines. It's a battle against time: if left untreated, the patient's leg weakness can progress to total paralysis within a few hours.

One of the eternal curiosities of radiation oncology practice is the arrival of patients with cord compression in clusters on Friday afternoon.

For this reason, many Rad Oncs dread being on call at the end of the week. One young, normally cheerful colleague became uncharacteristically irritable when he had five patients in various stages of cord compression arrive in a row late one Friday. The unpleasant truth behind "Friday afternoon syndrome" is the neglect of reports of scans done on patients earlier in the week. As he or she plows through a pile of accumulated lab reports before departing for the weekend, a doctor at another hospital suddenly notices an MRI done on Tuesday that showed a cord compression. This prompts a panicky phone call to the radiation doctor on call. Not only do such delays place pressure on the radiation department at the end of a busy work week but, more important, they place patients at high risk for deterioration. I've seen more than one patient who was able to move their legs at the time of the MRI but was completely paralysed by the time they came to see me a few days later. Numbness and loss of control of the sphincter muscles controlling bladder function follow weakness. It's a sad truth too that many of these patients have advanced cancer, and often their leg weakness is ascribed to "fatigue," and a possible cord compression is not considered until the damage is irreversible. New leg weakness in a cancer patient should always be investigated, and patients and families should be diligent about making sure test results are followed up.

On a weekend like today, the situation is complicated by the radiation department being closed, so I have to ask the on-call radiation therapists to come in, turn on the machines, and perform the detailed safety checks needed before any patient is treated. Many of the therapists are young and have small children, and calling them in causes greater impact on their personal lives than mine. My practice is to give them a warning call, a heads-up that I might need their help. On the way to the hospital today I've called Glenn, an enthusiastic young therapist who, in between shushing his kids, responds with his usual cheerful assurance that he'll be there as soon as I need him.

Many spinal cord compressions occur in patients already known to have metastatic cancer, so the news they have developed a new complication, while unwelcome, is not surprising. For these patients, a cord compression often heralds the terminal phase of their illness, especially if leg weakness leaves them with reduced mobility and bedridden, making them vulnerable to other complications such as blood clots and pneumonia. One challenge in these situations is avoiding over-radiation to areas of the spine that may have already received radiation to control pain or even to previous areas of cord compression. Like all organs in the body, there's a limit to the radiation dose a structure such as the spinal cord can absorb. Too much can cause damage, resulting in the very problem we're trying to prevent: paralysis. For these patients, further radiation may be impossible and surgery has to be considered, but often these patients are too sick for an operation and must be cared for with painkillers and other palliative manoeuvres.

For other patients, such as Mr. Singh, a cord compression is the first unwelcome manifestation of cancer. Patients and their families reel from both a frightening physical condition and the shock of an unexpected cancer diagnosis. And it's not just cancer: it's already advanced, metastatic, in the spine. The lifespan of most patients in this situation is limited to a few months, a few years if they are lucky enough to have a cancer that responds well to hormones or chemotherapy. As if this isn't distressing enough, there is the added uncertainty of making a diagnosis without a biopsy, on the clinical history and imaging results alone. All of this information has to be communicated somehow in the hurried, cramped confines of an emergency room cubicle. I understand Mr. Singh's son's shock and hesitancy.

"Radiation? Isn't there another option?"

"The ER already called the neurosurgeon on call. He looked at the scans and doesn't think an operation is possible."

"Why not?"

"For one thing, it's a huge operation that involves scraping out the diseased bone and replacing it with a kind of cement. Your dad has at least two areas that need operating. He's very frail, and the surgeon doesn't think he'd pull through it very well. Don't forget, surgery involves an anesthetic and the risk of infection."

"But radiation – that will make him sick."

"It will be focused on the areas where the cord is being compressed. He might get some redness on the skin of his back where the radiation goes in, and maybe a bit of trouble swallowing in a few days."

"Swallowing? Why?"

I indicate a collapsed tube running in front of the spine.

"This is the oesophagus, the swallowing tube. It will get irritated by the radiation. Shall we get on with it?'

The son looks at his father. "I'm not sure."

"The sooner we do it, the better. If we wait until your father is completely paralysed, it may be too late for him to recover."

"No. I want to talk to my older brother first. He's a doctor in the US."

He says "Doctor-in-the-US" like he belongs to some higher order of physicians, privy to secrets of medical lore we mere Canadians lack.

I feel a knot of irritation forming in my stomach. The phone call will cause more delay. I take a big breath and the knot loosens.

"What kind of doctor is he?"

"Dermatologist."

A dermatologist? He'll know as much about malignant spinal cord compression as I do about atopic dermatitis.

"Okay, go ahead, speak to him. In the meantime, can we give your father some medicine to control any secondary swelling in the spine?"

The son nods. He punches a number into his cell phone and retreats to a curtained recess on the far side of his father's stretcher.

I ask the nurse to give Mr. Singh an IV dose of a powerful steroid, dexamethasone. With any luck, it will prevent deterioration over the next couple of hours and buy some time. I retreat behind the counter and flop in a chair. I gaze at the slumped figures of patients on stretchers and wheelchairs around me. Backed by the incessant rhythm of beeping monitors, nurses dart between the forest of IV poles to attend to patients. I hear a moan of pain from a nearby cubicle; from another, the muffled sound of sobs. Death flutters from cubicle to cubicle, stretcher to stretcher, making rapid assessments. Cancer work is chaotic, but this is far worse.

Every now and then the main door of the emergency department slides open, unravelling a brief carpet of sunlight into the lobby and releasing a waft of sweet spring air, welcome relief from the foul odours around me.

Phone to his ear, Mr. Singh's son approaches. "It's my brother," he mouths, and hands me the phone.

"Good morning, it's Dr. Hayter."

"Dr. Hayter, how are you? It's Dr. Singh."

I briefly review the situation with the dermatologist, who, as I suspected, knows as little about spinal cord compressions as I do about the current treatment of psoriasis. Our conversation highlights the thick walls of the silos separating medical specialties. I simplify my explanation to the language understood by a first-year medical student.

At the end of each of my sentences he says, "Uh-huh," like a liturgical response. At the end, after I summarize my recommendations, there's a pause, then his voice takes an authoritative tone.

"So, doctor, you really want to give radiation without a tissue diagnosis?"

His tone now makes me feel like the student. "Once the radiation is done, we can arrange a biopsy of the lung mass."

He emits a harsh, slightly mocking laugh.

"Ha-ha. Sounds like you Canadians are a bit trigger-happy with radiation. Sorry, but I'm going to set up a second opinion for my dad down here."

"Where's that?"

"North Carolina."

I take a huge breath.

"Sir, there's no time for that. By the time he gets there he could be paralysed."

"I want my dad getting the best treatment possible."

Just then, the younger son gives a frantic wave from his father's bedside.

"Uh-oh. Something's happened to your dad. I'll have to call you back."

I move to the stretcher and hand the phone back.

"What's going on?"

The son points to a damp stain in the valley of the sheet between Mr. Singh's legs.

· I lift the wet sheet and pick up Mr. Singh's left leg. It's heavy, lifeless, a dead log lifted from the forest floor.

"Uh-oh. He's become incontinent. And his legs are much weaker."

I draw a small gadget, a flat metal wheel with spiky edges like a pizza cutter, from my pocket and roll it gently upwards along Mr. Singh's torso. When it reaches his belly button, he flinches.

"He's losing the sensation in the lower part of his body."

Cancer has a way of prodding situations along. The tumour is now pressing on the tracts carrying sensation from the lower limbs.

Death drifts closer and gives a thumbs-up of approval.

I stare hard at the son.

"His condition's deteriorating. There's no more time to waste. We have to do something now. Do you want your dad to get completely paralysed in front of your eyes?"

· The tension on his face dissolves. His lips quiver. He transforms into a schoolboy about to burst into tears.

"No. This can't be happening. Just when we brought him over from India to live with us."

"What about your mom?"

"She passed away last year."

"I'm sorry."

"He was looking forward to his new life with us. He was a farmer back home. He's planted a veggie garden in our backyard."

"He won't be able to garden if his legs don't work. I'm sorry, I never asked your name."

"Harpreet, sir."

Glenn, the radiation therapist on call, bounds through the swinging doors at the end of the ER.

At his entrance, Death recoils and retreats behind an IV stand.

"Morning! Ready to go. The machine's all warmed up."

"This is Glenn, the on-call radiation therapist. He's going to take your dad away and set up the treatment. Okay?"

"Okay," Harpreet mumbles.

Glenn kicks the brakes of Mr. Singh's stretcher, starts to push him away, then stops and turns. "Wait. Where's the consent?"

Shit. I forgot. Glenn is bound by hospital rules not to start any treatment until he's seen proof the patient has given consent.

I move towards the head of Mr. Singh's stretcher.

"I have to speak to your father."

"He only speaks Punjabi," says Harpreet.

"Can you translate?"

"Uh ... no."

"He has to understand the situation and give his consent."

"I don't want him knowing anything about what's going on."

"Then I'll have to call a translator."

I reach to the phone on the desk. Harpreet grabs my arm.

"Please, no."

He tightens his grip. A band of pain wraps around my biceps. I feel a surge of anger at what amounts to a physical assault. I pull myself away and take another big breath.

Glenn steps forward with his signature sunny grin.

"Sir. We can't give radiation until we know your father understands the reason for it and has said yes."

"It will just upset him and make him sicker. Just go ahead and do what you have to do. I give my consent."

"That's not enough," Glenn says, glancing at me. "Do you have a power of attorney for your father's care?"

"What's that?"

"A document signed by your father to say you can make decisions about his medical care."

"I told you, he's never been sick. Why would I have that?"

"Then I have to talk to him," I say.

It's an all too familiar situation. Some families work hard to erect a seemingly impregnable barrier of denial around elderly relatives. It's an extension of the curtain of silence dropped around the word cancer. I've often been ambushed by adult children in the corridor as I make my way towards an examining room, before I've even clapped eyes on their parent with cancer. With one patient, a gaggle of middle-aged daughters rushed at me, waving their arms, shouting, "Doctor! Please don't tell Mama she has cancer. It will kill her!"

What's behind this behaviour? As in Harpreet's case, it usually stems from a desire to protect the parent from the pain of distressing news and from the misguided idea it will somehow make the cancer worse. In my experience it transcends cultural boundaries and arises from individual family dynamics and communication styles. In some families, painful subjects such as death, serious illness, crime, or sexual diversity are just off limits for discussion. I've seen this just as often in well-heeled WASP families as in immigrant Asian families.

It places me and the staff in a difficult situation. For at least the past fifty years, informed consent has been a cornerstone of medical practice. It arose in response to shameful episodes in medical history when doctors performed experiments or novel treatments on unsuspecting patients without their knowledge and often to their harm. The most famous example is the Tuskegee experiments, in which treatment was deliberately withheld from Black men with syphilis. Informed consent requires that before proceeding with treatment, I explain the diagnosis, proposed treatment, and side effects to the patient, and answer all questions to their satisfaction. Obtaining and documenting consent has become part of the normal process prior to any medical procedure and is even more important prior to a poorly understood and potentially harmful treatment such as radiation. The only circumstance where it can be waived is an emergency in which immediate action must be taken to preserve life. Spinal cord compression is an emergency but it does not directly threaten life.

Efforts to deke around consent make things difficult for the patient too. Bad news is bound to upset, but there is no evidence it leads to depression and the loss of hope. On the contrary, the truth allows patients to understand their situation and set realistic expectations about their future. It begins the process of creating realistic hopes. Without knowing the truth, the patient will be plunged into bewilderment and fear – potentially a worse kind of anguish than confronting the truth.

Glenn, Harpreet, and I stand in a silent triangle at the head of Mr. Singh's stretcher, gazing at the old man's face. Death peers at us from his alcove.

The father looks small, alone, afraid. His eyes dart between us. What is he thinking? *Why have my legs become useless? Why am I here in this crowded, noisy emergency department? Why did I have that scan? What did it show?* And if he proceeds to radiation: *Why am I being taken to a department called "Cancer Centre?" Do I have cancer? Why is nobody telling me? Why am I being strapped to this table? Why are those thin red lights aimed at my flanks? Why are they pointing that huge machine at my back? What's going on?*

Surely the truth is better than these confusing questions.

I've got to give him radiation. It's his only chance to avoid total paralysis. He has terminal cancer, but I don't want him to spend the rest of his days bedridden.

Various scenarios unfold in my mind. I can't just abandon him. I could ask Harpreet to leave, call an interpreter, and interview Mr. Singh on my own. But this would likely leave Harpreet thwarted and angry.

In situations like this, it's always important for me to think clearly and remember two principles: first, legally, my only responsibility is to the patient, and not to the family, no matter how forceful its members are. Second, I am not compelled legally or ethically to give information to someone who has expressed a clear preference not to know it. A competent patient can waive the right to receive information.

This last approach offers a way out of the impasse. It doesn't escalate the situation, and it puts the patient, Mr. Singh, and not his sons, in control.

"I understand your concern, but at the very least I need to know how much your dad wants to know," I say. "If he says he doesn't want to be involved, then that's fine, we can proceed. Can you at least ask your dad how much he wants to know?"

Harpreet hesitates, then goes to his dad's side, leans over, and says something in Punjabi. I just have to trust that his words are an accurate translation of my question.

Mr. Singh briefly raises his head and stares at me. His eyes glint briefly like crystals in a cave. His lips curve into a gentle smile. His expression is slightly mischievous, as if to say, *Don't mind my son. Just humour him. I know very well what's going on.*

It's like a flip of the situation in a family of a gay person, when parents know a child is gay but the child continues to deny or conceal it. "Honey, we always knew," the parents chortle, after the child finally comes out.

Harpreet turns back to me.

"I told him there's a problem in his spine and this doctor's going to help you. He says good, you look like a nice doctor. He trusts you to just go ahead and do what you need to do. I'll call my brother back and tell him there's no need for a second opinion."

Part of me wants to demand he tell his father the whole truth right here and now, but there's no time for further bickering. There will be plenty of time for honest discussions in the coming days.

"Good to go," says Glenn, and wheels the stretcher towards the door. Propped up on pillows, Mr. Singh glides regally past the rows of waiting patients, pressed palms raised in silent *namaste*. Death throws up his hands and turns to busy himself with other patients.

A month later, Mr. Singh returns to see me in the outpatient clinic. Since I saw him, he's finished radiation to his spine with very few side effects. He's also had a biopsy of the tumour in his lung, which confirms he has lung cancer.

The good news is that it is a subtype of lung cancer that can be kept under control by chemotherapy. He's already seen a medical oncologist and has received his first dose of chemo.

For me, the best news of all is that the cancer in his spine has responded very well to radiation, so he's resumed his early morning walks and has been able to continue working on his veggie patch.

Harpreet hands me a crumpled brown paper bag.

"My dad grew these. He wants to say thank you."

I tug the bag open and a rich loamy scent emerges. Inside, there's a cluster of plump juicy carrots, still moist and dusty from the soil.

9

The Pushy Patient

In any case, my father doesn't need my meddling. He already has someone by his side who won't hesitate to interfere if necessary.

If my strategy to connect with my father was to become a Doctor, my mother's was to become a Patient.

For as long as I remember, she complained of ill health. A cursory review of letters written to me over decades shows a list of ailments ranging from "crushed vertebrae," "wasted muscles," "suspicious moles," through recalcitrant "bugs in the urine," to more ominous conditions such as "internal haemorrhages," "heart trouble," and even "leukemia." Her eyes, thyroid, sinuses, and bowels gave her endless trouble. Never satisfied with one diagnosis, she spent a great deal of time, energy, and money rushing to appointments with specialists and having scans of different parts of her body. Her nursing background gave her a thorough medical vocabulary, useful for quelling the sceptics.

Eventually, her illnesses coalesced into a self-diagnosis of systemic lupus, an autoimmune disease known as the "great imitator" because its symptoms can mimic those of many other conditions. Her myriad complaints, from double vision to ulcers to a "poorly functioning liver," could be conveniently gathered under one rubric. Lupus gets its name from the Latin word for wolf because its characteristic butterfly-shaped facial rash looks like a wolf's bite. My mother never exhibited this rash. From my review of her extant medical records, there was never any firm evidence she suffered from lupus. Nonetheless, she persevered. The diagnosis afforded her not only a tidy package for her complaints but also a succinct shield for emotional protection: "Don't upset me, it'll make my lupus act up!" When the wolf flared, my siblings and I crept around, afraid of provoking it. No letter to me was complete without a report, often tinged with melodrama, on her lupus. "It is fatal, I will always have guts and fight on," she wrote, decades before she died.

Despite the flimsy if non-existent evidence for her diagnosis, my father never challenged it. Not confrontational by nature, he silently colluded, partly, I suppose, out of his devotion to her, partly out of fear of her wrath. My mother's temper sometimes exploded in fits of shrieking and hurling crockery across the front hall as he beat a quick exit. He signed a certificate enabling her to get a permit to park in spots designated for the disabled. At the hospital, he worked with technicians called prosthetists, staff skilled in the crafting of artificial limbs and other devices to help the disabled. From their workshop, he brought home a steady stream of gadgets for my mother's use, the most terrifying of which was a cane with a retractable claw at the end. In my mother's hand, it became a weapon to scare away unwelcome dogs or children, or to intimidate unhelpful department store sales staff.

My mother conducted her life costumed in her wolf clothing and assisted by such props. In Canada, her English accent, which she modulated from barmaid Cockney to regal dulcet depending on the situation, gave her an extra weapon. As she shoved herself to the front of queues in department stores or at airline counters, she morphed into a frightening – and to her children, always embarrassing – version of the British Battleaxe, an even more boisterous, volatile, confrontational version of Hyacinth Bucket.

We forgave her antics partly because, like Mrs. Bucket, she possessed a zest for life, a sense of humour, and could, when the mood was right, be outrageously jolly. She loved organizing parties, outings, and picnics. In keeping with her innate English pluck, weather never deterred an outing. At a tailgate picnic in Banff we stood shivering in the mountain air as we chomped on tuna sandwiches on which snowflakes were settling. She had a special enthusiasm for parlour games and often enlivened otherwise dreary gatherings of my father's colleagues by distributing papers and pencils for spontaneous and sometimes incomprehensible "quizzes."

We also sensed a deep sadness behind the masks she wore, a sadness likely caused by the abrupt wrench from her homeland and extended family when we moved to Canada, and also by some unhappy experiences of bullying in childhood. During my teenage years in Winnipeg, she disappeared on occasion into the hospital, where I later learned she received electroconvulsive therapy – then a conventional treatment for even mild depression. And her bathroom cabinet was always well stocked with tranquilizers my father smuggled from the hospital.

My mother's manipulative use of illness left me with a scepticism of medical complaints; not a flattering quality in a doctor. Throughout my medical career I've had to guard against suspecting patients of faking symptoms. I've also always been more than a little scared of Pushy Patients.

"What time is my treatment?"

The voice of the patient, a seventy-year-old retired judge with early stage prostate cancer, booms from the centre of the examining room. He's a tall, heavyset man whose imposing figure and angry frown elicits a flutter of anxiety in my belly, a feeling such as must have been felt by many a witness or attorney in his courtroom.

I glance nervously at the wall separating us from the patient in the next room.

"Would you mind keeping your voice down?" I ask.

"When is it?" he thunders.

"Well, uh, it's not today ..." I stammer.

"Tomorrow then?"

"It's not so simple. There's a few steps before you start."

"Steps? What kind of steps?" The thunder claps louder.

"Well, first I need to take a history –"

"It's all there," he barks, indicating his file on my desk.

"Yes, but I'd like to review it with you to make sure it's accurate. Why don't you sit down?"

"Sit down. Why?"

He takes a threatening step towards me, and his belly eclipses all the objects in the room. Lines from Shakespeare's "seven ages of man" speech appear in my head: "the justice, in fair round belly with good capon lined." I can't help imagining all the good capon packed inside this belly.

"Please give me a minute."

I swivel to my desk and open his file. He snorts.

"Christ, what a bloody waste of time. I'll be late for my round of golf."

I quickly flip through his file. Like the vast majority of men with prostate cancer, his cancer came to light from an elevated PSA. A urologist performed biopsies that showed cancer in the prostate. Scans showed no evidence of metastases.

"Okay, from what I can see you've got curable prostate cancer. Are you having any symptoms?"

"I already told the nurse. No."

"Please lie down on the couch."

"Why?"

"I need to examine you."

"Christ. I came here to get radiation, not to get fingered."

He carries a common misconception. He assumes I'm some kind of technician whose job is simply to slot him in for radiation. He doesn't know radiation oncologists are medical doctors who, like every other doctor, must begin every assessment with a history and physical. Then, we formulate our own opinion of whether radiation is appropriate.

"Please lie on the table and unbuckle your pants."

"Nobody's sticking their finger up my ass again."

I muster a weak smile.

"I'm sorry, I'm a doctor, and I really can't arrange anything further for you until I've checked you for myself."

He glares, then heaves himself onto the examining table and unbuckles his belt.

"Okay, but make it quick."

"Please turn, and pull the back of your pants down"

He rolls to his left and slides his pants down. A shower of coins spills from his pockets and clatters to the floor. I crouch and gather the shiny discs. Maybe a joke will help.

"Was that my tip?"

· He scowls at me over his shoulder.

I place the handful of coins on the desk and turn back to him. A pair of large pink buttocks, smooth and shiny as party balloons, pop from the gap between the bottom of his shirt and his belt.

I slip on a pair of latex gloves, anoint the tip of my right index finger with lubricating gel, and gently spread his buttocks with the fingers of my left hand.

He clenches his anus tightly.

"Hell. I don't know how those gay guys do this."

I suppress a strong urge to jab him.

"Just relax. Relax, please. Take a big breath. Big breath."

He hisses in air through clenched teeth, his anus relaxes, and my finger slides in. He writhes and emits an unexpectedly high-pitched pig-like squeal.

"Jesus."

"I'll just be a second."

I quickly sweep my finger around the rectum, searching for the contour of the prostate. There it is, at the front, a soft, spongy gland the size of a small tangerine. It's clearly enlarged: I suspect he's not telling the truth when he says he has no symptoms. And there, on the right side, corresponding to where the biopsy showed cancer, my finger encounters a stony-hard lump, a pebble in a pudding. Compared to other prostate cancers, such as Peter's, it's very small.

"Oh yes, there's a nodule."

"What? Nobody told me that."

I quickly withdraw my finger and toss the gloves in the can.

"You can sit up."

His immense form rolls and sits. A sheen of moisture covers his forehead. I offer him a box of tissues, but he waves it away.

"Dr. Little sent you here for an opinion about radiation. I think it would be a good option for you. For your stage of cancer, it's equivalent to surgery."

"Yah, yah, I've done my homework. I know all this. Let's get on with it.'

"Great. I'll book you for planning."

"What's that?"

"To get you ready for treatment. It involves a special CT scan."

"Christ, I just had a CT."

Misconception number two: a patient can proceed directly to radiation without preparation steps.

"That was a diagnostic scan. This is a different CT, to map out the prostate so the beams can be aimed accurately."

"Today?"

"No. In two, three days."

"My treatment starts that day?"

"Perhaps a week after."

His jaw works and bubbles of saliva trickle from the corners of his lips.

"Jesus. The urologist told me this would be a piece of cake."

"I'm afraid other doctors are sometimes not aware of what's involved in giving radiation."

Ignorance like this always reminds me of a survey showing that very few medical schools offer exposure to radiation oncology to students.

"I want this over and done with. I got a cruise booked for the end of the month."

"Hmmm. There's no way we can get everything – planning, treatment – done before then. Sorry – you'd better look into rebooking."

"Impossible."

I think of the glacial delays in the judicial system. How would he respond if I jumped up and down in court asking for a trial to be concluded today? I glance at my watch and move towards the door.

"Oops, I'm running behind. Look, I'll get you in the system as quickly as I can. Please wait here. Kim will come and explain the procedure from here on. Nice to meet you. Oh – don't forget those."

I indicate the pile of coins on the desk, resist a strong urge to bow, then dart quickly through the door and into the workroom. I toss the file on the desk, take a big breath, and twist my knuckles into my temples.

Kim, the cheery, unflappable nurse on duty with me today, glances at me. "Ah – a Rosedale Special?"

Rosedale is a leafy, affluent district of immense mansions and sweeping gardens in central Toronto. "Rosedale Special" is our secret code for a difficult, demanding patient whose sense of entitlement leads to requests for special treatment.

"The King."

Kim likes nothing more than to take a Special on. Girding herself with an armful of educational pamphlets about prostate cancer, she marches towards the judge's chamber.

"Good luck," I call after her.

I must initiate arrangements for the judge's treatment by first filling out a requisition. I sit at the computer, draw open the curtains to my electronic playhouse, and pull up the judge's file. In addition to the boxes for Curative and Palliative, the banner at the top of the page has a button marked Urgency that, when pressed, releases a drop-down menu of options that floats over the screen like scenery descending from the flies in an eighteenth-century playhouse. Like the intent of treatment, my choice of urgency is essential for the staff to make bookings for the patient. Emergency is for patients with life- or organ-threatening problems such as spinal cord compression who must receive treatment the same day as being seen by me. Urgent is for those patients with symptoms such as bleeding or breathlessness whose treatment must be started quickly, within three or four days. Everyone else – the vast majority of patients, whether receiving radiation prior to surgery, after surgery, or as definitive treatment – is marked Routine, which means starting within fourteen days of being seen by me. To an outsider, fourteen days may seem a long time, but it's not wasted: the preparation of the treatment plan, particularly for patients receiving a high dose, where care must be taken to protect healthy tissues, is a lengthy and complicated process involving multiple handoffs and quality checks between medical, radiotherapy, and physics staff.

I place a check in the box beside Curative. That's easy. But the choice of urgency is more difficult. My cursor hovers over the drop-down menu. His medical circumstances dictate the Routine fourteen-day urgency, but his thunderous tones ring in my ears. I'm tempted to mark his case Urgent. Sometimes, under pressure by patients or families, or because of compassion for a particular patient's circumstances, I've stretched the definition of Urgent to include patients who otherwise could wait for two weeks. My colleagues and I sometimes make personal appeals to the staff to get patients on treatment as early as possible in that two-week window.

But a cruise? It's hard to muster compassion for a high-end vacation. Plus he's annoyed me enough already that I feel compelled to dig in my heels a bit. Prostate cancer is slow-growing, and delaying a patient's treatment will have no effect on the outcome. I click the Routine fourteen-day option and send the requisition to the booking staff.

If you wander into the treatment area of a modern radiation clinic, you're likely to find yourself in a long dark corridor lined with entrances to the "bunkers" containing the treatment machines. It's a bit like entering a vast ancient mausoleum lined with doorways opening to dimly lit vaults. Each of these vaults contains a mighty machine, a linear accelerator (linac), a device of ingenious engineering capable of creating beams of potentially lethal radiation. Such is the power of these machines that the primary beam creates secondary photons that bounce and ricochet in all directions, requiring the machines to be enclosed in concrete walls and only accessed by a twisting maze – adding to the feeling that one is entering a hidden funeral chamber. Most bunkers are designed to keep danger out; ours are designed to keep danger in.

Linacs are the culmination of radiotherapy's quest to develop machines with ever increasing penetration. In the early years of the twentieth century, external radiotherapy was given by clunky "deep-X-ray units" whose beams could penetrate only a few centimetres beneath the skin. Their use was restricted by painful blistering-skin reactions. One such machine may be glimpsed in the 1993 film *Shadowlands*, about C.S. Lewis's wife's diagnosis and death from cancer. In some medical quarters, "DXR" lingers as shorthand for radiotherapy. In the 1950s, a Canadian invention, the cobalt unit, supplanted X-ray units. Its beams, generated from a source of radioactive cobalt, were far more penetrating than X-rays and spared the skin. Finally, cobalt units gave way to linacs, which produce beams of such intensity that even the most deeply seated cancers can be treated. Linacs are now the mainstay of every radiation department worldwide – although some developing countries still use cobalt machines, since their operation is simpler.

Linacs are big, complicated machines with, like every other piece of hospital equipment, a finite capacity. In most hospitals, these big machines operate for around nine hours a day, with each machine treating about 25 patients in that time. In a department with six machines, the total daily throughput – to use an ugly bureaucratic term reminiscent of a sausage factory – is thus about 150 patients.

In an ideal world, these 150 slots would exactly match the number of patients requiring treatment, and, apart from the interval required to prepare the treatment, there would be no waiting. As soon as the treatment plan is prepared, a patient could zip to a vacant spot on a machine. But it's not so simple. In recent decades, the number of cancer cases and the number of patients requiring radiation has risen inexorably year by year. This phenomenon is caused by multiple factors, including an aging population, an absolute rise in certain types of cancer, and expansion of the uses of radiation to treat cancer. As a result, there is always a queue of patients snaking from my clinic to the linacs via the planning and preparation area.

The solution seems easy: install new machines to increase capacity. But each new linac costs approximately C$2 million and requires construction of its own expensive bunker. Capital costs aside, there's also the ongoing operational costs of staffing and maintenance.

In Ontario, the radiation capacity crisis of the 1980s resulted in both shorter dose schedules and improvements in the organization of radiation departments, which included introduction of the urgency categories that now float down daily on my drop-down menu. The dates are carefully monitored to ensure patients' first appointments don't slip beyond two weeks from the initial appointment with me. In addition to my other roles, I'm now the ticket agent who determines in what class the patient travels.

The next morning, I'm upstairs in my private cubbyhole, swigging coffee and scanning accumulated emails. My eye falls on one marked "Urgent."

Dr. Hayter:
Bad news. Treatment Appointment Monday November 6th.
Unacceptable. Please change.
Justice Otis McNichol, LLD, QC

I almost sputter coffee on the keyboard. How did this guy get my private hospital email address, used only for internal correspondence about patients and administrative matters?

I open his file and look up his calendar of appointments. Monday, November 6th is two weeks from yesterday, the day I first saw him. His treatment is booked to start right at the end of the acceptable fourteen-day waiting interval for a non-urgent case. He's been seated in the last row of the third-class carriage, but he'll still arrive at an acceptable time.

On my way downstairs, I peer into the tiny carrel occupied by Lesley, our friendly, organized administrative assistant, whose head is always buried in a pile of patient files.

"Morning. By any chance, did you give my email address to a patient?"
Lesley's lips curve down into a pout, and she stares at me.

"I would never do that."

"Okay. Funny. I got an email direct from a patient this morning."

"Oh, I wonder if it's the same guy that's been calling. McNichol?"

"That's the one."

"Left me two voice messages about his appointment. I haven't had time to call him back."

"Leave it with me. I'll get back to him."

Uh-oh. I sense trouble ahead with the judge. Sometimes there's wiggle room within the two-week window, caused by cancellations or changes in a patient's treatment, and occasionally appointments can be brought forward. I decide to pay a visit to the Keeper of the Waiting List, Sheila, the assistant manager of the radiation department. She's a poker-faced, slightly fierce Scot, with hair twisted to short spiky black bristles. Sheila's job is slotting patients into treatment slots according to urgency. She guards against tampering with the list with the doggedness of a dragon guarding a cave stacked with treasure. But sometimes, if I ask nicely ...

I peer sheepishly around her door.

"Morning, Sheila," I say with a bright smile.

"Morning," she says, her eyes not lifting from her screen. "If it's about pushing McNichol up, there's nothing I can do."

"Oh – you know about him?"

"He called me direct. I just got off the phone with him. I told him we're fully booked."

"How did he take it?"

"Hung up on me."

Poor Sheila. How does she cope with such rudeness? It's not the first time she's been harassed by an anxious patient or by a persistent doctor who wants his or her patient moved up.

"Nothing you can do for him?"

She fixes her small emerald eyes on me.

"Things are so bad, we may need to go to extended hours."

Extended hours. The term is enough to send a shiver up my spine. Every now and then, in response to a surge in patients, the hours of operation of the linacs are extended to accommodate extra patients who might otherwise fall outside the two-week limit. These surges are unpredictable and seem to be tied to the seasons. Because radiation oncologists depend mostly on surgeons for referrals, there is always a drop in referrals during the holiday periods of the summer and around Christmas, followed by a burst of referrals in the weeks after, when the surgeons are back at work. Although everyone knows it's to benefit patients, the term "extended hours" is enough to send a rumble of discontent through the radiation department. The therapists, many of whom are young and have small children, will have to juggle their childcare responsibilities, and the doctors will have to arrange on-call coverage for the extra hours. The last time this happened, when the hours were increased from nine per day to twelve, staff started to look weary, and a sense of impending burnout hovered over the department. It's hard enough for the radiation therapists to be face to face with cancer patients for nine hours. Those in the upper floors of the hospital who make decisions about extended hours do not recognize the emotional impact of working with cancer patients day in and day out.

Sheila has better things to do than deal with me. I feel bad about my temptation to harass her, and take my leave.

I hear nothing further from the judge, so I assume Sheila's call has placated him. He gets his planning CT done that day, and the next morning I'm sitting at the computer, gazing at the images of the interior of his belly in preparation for outlining his target volume. Under the vast sweeping arch of his tummy, I spot his plump kidneys, his twisted, bloated bowel, and – ha-ha – is that an undigested capon over there? I locate his prostate, a grey blob wedged between his rectum and bladder, and begin outlining it.

I'm halfway through contouring the prostate when the phone rings. It's Lesley.

"There's a call for you."

"I'm tied up. Can you ask them to call back?"

"I think you'd better take it. It's one of the VPs."

A VP of the hospital? Why would he or she want to get in touch with me? Lesley connects us.

"Morning, Dr. Hayter," chirps a bright female voice with the enthusiastic tone of a morning radio-show host. "It's Sandy from development."

"Hello?"

Sandy? Sandy? Oh yes, the VP of development for the hospital. I remember her from a hospital fundraiser at which doctors like me were trotted out to meet and impress prospective donors. I recall a short trim figure, who stomped from group to group on gleaming black stilettoes, flashing a brilliant white smile at everyone.

"How's your day going?"

"Fine."

"Great. I just had a call from Justice McNichol. Isn't he a wonderful guy?"

"Uh, yuh."

"He tells me there's going to be a wait before he can start his treatment."

"Only a week or so."

Her tone becomes confidential. "You should know something. He's a very generous donor to the hospital."

"Uh-huh?"

"There's a couple of upcoming capital projects we're counting on his support for. In fact, we're planning on naming a building after him."

I feel queasy at the thought of arriving at the hospital in the future to see this man's name permanently etched on the side of a building.

"Is there anything you can do to squeeze him in earlier?"

"Not really. Our machines are at full capacity."

I suppress the urge to remind her that a couple of years back, the Radiation Department had submitted a proposal to her for a capital campaign to raise money for new equipment to ease the backlog of patients. The proposal was rejected in favour of some new fancy cardiac equipment. In the beauty contest of hospital fundraising, heart often wins over cancer.

"I'm sure there must be something you can do."

"It's not so easy ..."

"I'm counting on you. Have a great day." There's a click as she hangs up.

There's nothing I can do to advance the judge's appointment. But he doesn't give up. Over the next few days, he sends a relentless stream of messages to me, Kim, Lesley, and Sheila, asking for a change in his appointment. Every time we check our emails or voicemails, there he is. He's playing the ancient game of water torture with us. He's hoping the relentless drip of calls and messages will wear us down.

At the end of the week, I'm halfway through a follow-up clinic of more than twenty patients, performing my typical waltz between rooms, examining patients and dispensing good, bad, or ambiguous news. As I emerge into the corridor from an examining room where I've just delivered bad news about a follow-up scan to a man with a brain tumour, an immense dark figure looms at the end of the corridor.

It's the judge. Arms folded across his chest, he glares like a detective interrogating a suspect.

"You," he bellows. "This is your last chance."

"Uh, I'm tied up seeing patients."

"Why has nothing been done about my appointment?"

He takes a step towards me. Kim darts from a side door and blocks his path.

"Sir, you can't come in here without an appointment," she says with a cheery but forceful tone. "Please go outside."

"I'm not going anywhere until my appointment's been changed."

I indicate an empty examining room.

"Okay. Why don't you come in here and we can talk for a minute?"

Kim's eyes flash. She doesn't like the flow of a clinic being interrupted. "You're already running behind."

"Give us a minute."

The judge lumbers after me into the room, and I close the door.

"Have a seat."

"No. So why hasn't anything been done?"

Actor's training again. I plant my feet firmly on the floor, square my shoulders, and look him straight in the eyes.

"I'm sorry. You'll have to wait your turn."

"Bullshit. There's got to be something you can do."

"You spoke to the manager, Sheila. I'm sure she told you patients go on the treatment machines in the order I've seen them. It's just not fair to push you to the head of the line."

"Come on. I'm sure there's someone who's less urgent than me who can wait."

"The system just doesn't work that way."

His cheeks puff and turn purple. I'm afraid his head might pop off. Dark stains creep from under his arms and from the creases of his shirt beneath his belly. The room fills with the odour of stale deodorant.

As we stare at each other in silent standoff, an image of the polite, soft-spoken pastor, a recent immigrant from Nigeria, whom I saw the same day as the judge, comes to mind. He had a similarly early curable prostate cancer and has also been booked for radiation. He's at home, patiently biding his time, waiting for his turn on the machine without complaint. I think of all the other voiceless patients, many of whose first language isn't English, who are patiently waiting. Why should I give this entitled blatherskite preference over the others?

"You're talking to me like I'm waiting for a limo at the airport. This isn't a goddamn taxi ride. I'm dealing with goddamn c ... c ... cancer."

His voice cracks. His eyes glisten. His belly quivers.

"You have no idea what this is like. The wait is killing me."

For the first time, I glimpse the small, frightened man inside the hulk. I lay a hand on his shoulder.

"I understand. Who's at home with you?" I ask.

"My wife, of course," he snaps.

"Perhaps you should talk it over with her."

"No. She doesn't know about this."

"Oh. You haven't told your wife you have cancer?"

"Why should I?"

"It can help to have someone to talk to."

"I can get through this on my own."

He's not just scared: he's lonely and isolated.

"Perhaps I'll have you speak to one of our social workers."

"Social worker? What the hell for?"

"To help you cope."

"I am coping! I don't need to talk to some sissy social worker. I just ... I just want this over and done with."

"Everyone does. But to put things in perspective, the wait for your treatment is short compared with the waits before you saw me."

I remind him that it took two months between the detection of the elevated PSA and the initial meeting with the urologist, and then another month to get the biopsy done. All this time, long before he saw me, he was living with untreated cancer – a cancer that in all likelihood had been present for months, maybe years. Compared to other sectors of the health system, the Radiation Department is a wonder of efficiency.

The small, frightened man disappears behind the reinflating form of the judge. He draws himself up and stares down with the imperious look he must have used in the courtroom.

"Okay, doctor. Are you positive this delay won't do me any harm?"

"I think so."

"You *think* so. I want you to *know* so. What's the evidence my cancer won't get worse?"

"Well, uh, if you want the exact evidence, I'll have to look it up."

"Just as I thought. How the hell did I end up with a doctor who doesn't know what he's doing?"

Holy. I've tried compassion. I've tried reason. This is what I get in return?

Something snaps inside me. I'm tempted to do something I've never done before: run. I swivel to the door.

"Uhh ... I've got other patients waiting."

"I'm through with you. I'm going to take this into my own hands."

I stop. Uh-oh. I anticipate another, more fraught call from Sandy, from the hospital CEO, or even a politician pal of his.

"I've got a place in Florida. There's a hospital close by with a fantastic cancer centre. I called them. They promised to get me in lickety-split."

Ah, the good old USA. From the perspective of a state-run system like ours, it's a fantasy land where getting radiation is as easy as strolling into a fast-food restaurant and ordering up a hamburger. That is, if you've got the bucks or plenty of insurance.

"Are you sure? I mean, everything's arranged here."

"So long."

He pushes past me, yanks open the door, and lumbers off down the corridor.

As I watch his receding form, I can't help emitting a sigh of relief. I shouldn't be glad about a patient walking away, but I am. It's not as if, like Peter, he's abandoning treatment. If the judge has the resources to get his treatment elsewhere, bully for him. And – presto! – he's just opened a slot for another patient.

Kim sidles up to me.

"So, did you talk him into sticking with his appointment?"

"Nope. Guess what? He's off to the USA."

She smiles.

"I'll let Sheila know to take him off our list." She thrusts a file at me. "You're behind. Here's your next patient."

In the quiet of my office, I have to admit the judge's question about the possible harmful effects of delay is reasonable, and it niggles at me. Is waiting for radiotherapy, as my former mentor Dr. William Mackillop described it in the title of a provocative paper, also "killing time"?

Despite the eagle-eyed management of the waiting list by managers like Sheila, who carefully match patients' urgency with the available slots, I and my colleagues live with unspoken anxiety that maybe, just maybe, a patient's cancer will get worse while they wait to start. Cancer cells multiply and tumours grow, and theoretically, the longer they remain unchecked, the greater the risk of spread and seeding in other organs. Over time, a patient's condition can progress from curable localized to incurable widespread cancer. The idea of progression is the basis of screening for cancer in healthy individuals: early in their development, cancers are small enough to be detected at a curable stage.

Obvious cancer growth between my first assessment and the first treatment is rare but does happen. The radiation therapists have sometimes summoned me urgently to a linac, where I find them hunched over their monitors, gazing in perplexity at an unruly blob of lung cancer that's already breached the confines of the borders of the intended radiation area – borders sometimes set by me only a few days earlier. The therapists unbuckle the patient from the treatment couch and lead them to a side room for a difficult, fraught conversation with me about the cancer's growth. Then there is further delay as the entire treatment is replanned for the bigger cancer. I've seen similar situations with cancer on the outside of the body – such as a man with a corona of squamous cancer bursting from his forehead which, by the time he reached his radiation appointment, was starting to drip down his cheek like candle wax. His cancer was advancing so rapidly I quickly arranged for him to receive a single, swift blast of radiation to stun it while the first treatment plan could be revised. These situations and the delays they bring about from revising the treatment only inflame the anxieties of both patients and staff.

Such anecdotes aside, is there any scientific data showing harmful effects of delays on the outcome of treatment? Does waiting reduce the chance of cure? Researchers have only become interested in the topic in recent years. Traditionally, doctors have been far more attracted to more glamourous areas of study such as testing new and exciting treatments than sifting through reams of administrative data looking for correlations between appointment dates and outcomes.

Undoubtedly, the credit for placing delays in radiotherapy on a scientific footing belongs to Mackillop and his team at the Radiation Research Unit at Queen's University, Kingston. Just as Gordon Richards gave the clinical practice of radiotherapy a scientific basis in the 1930s, so too in the 1990s did Mackillop and his colleagues bring science to bear on the neglected epidemiological aspects of radiotherapy. His investigations, prompted largely by the Canadian waiting-list imbroglios of the 1980s, raised awareness of the problem of waiting times. His analysis showed that waits had risen inexorably, and also showed a vast discrepancy in waiting times between radiation centres. Since then, studies have shown that delay in radiotherapy undoubtedly affects the results of treatment for certain cancers. For the two most commonly studied cancers, head and neck and breast cancer, long delays before starting treatment can affect both control of the local cancer and survival.

But the effect of delay depends on the growth rate of a cancer. Different cancers progress at different rates. For rapidly growing cancers, such as the lung cancer whose growth caused consternation among the radiation therapists, even a short delay might affect outcome. For slow-growing cancers, such as the judge's prostate cancer, it's unlikely a delay of even a few weeks will change the prognosis. My attitude is supported by one study showing that waiting longer than two-and-a-half months between diagnosis and radiotherapy had no impact for patients with less-aggressive prostate cancers, although it did produce an unfavourable outcome for those with more aggressive cancers. The judge has a non-aggressive form of prostate cancer, so I am confident that a wait of a few days is not going to reduce his chance of cure.

None of this is to dismiss the emotional burden of waiting. The notion of sitting at home with untreated cancer for even two weeks, waiting for the phone to ring with an appointment, is scary at best. There will always be delay owing to the time it takes to prepare the treatment, but to quote the ASARA principle articulated by Mackillop: "Delays in radiotherapy should be As Short As Reasonably Achievable."

A week later, Lesley patches a call through to me.

"Dr. Hayter? It's McNichol," he bellows.

"Oh, hi. How are things in Florida?"

"Hot as hell. I, uh, need to ask you something ..."

"Uh-huh?"

"Seems things don't work down here as fast as I thought. They can't start my treatment for a week. Any way you can give me back my appointment at your place?"

10

The Fractured Family

My father receives ten radiation treatments to his spine.

My young hotshot's antipathy to this approach melts when I read my mother's description of the experience: the cancer centre is a "very nice place" where "every day we are served tea, coffee, ginger ale or juice and a plate of cookies (several varieties) on a doilied plate!! Drinks served in beautiful English bone china cups and saucers and a silver cream and sugar set!!"

My mother likes nothing better than being treated like royalty. I see her sipping tea and regaling her waiting-room neighbours with stories of her nursing days or her own afflictions from lupus. The friendliness, efficiency, and concern of the radiation staff impress my parents. Their daily visits provide an opportunity for socialization and support.

Through their experience, I see radiation from the perspective of a patient, and I reconsider my enthusiasm for a single dose. If it's convenient and comfortable for the patient, it may be better for their social and psychological well-being to come for multiple visits rather than the anonymous, wham-bam single shot I favoured. I carry this idea forward into my future practice.

By the spring of 1990, with the combination of the hormone-blocker pill and radiation to his spine, my father feels better. Best of all, his pain improves to the point he resumes daily walks with Tessie around a reservoir near their house. Some days, inhaling deep lungfuls of the fresh spring air, he even jogs part way. He putters again in the garden and his basement hideaway. In confirmation of the improvement, repeat X-rays show the ivory densities in his spine to be shrunk, blurry, dissolving.

As the weeks and months go by, and the news from Calgary becomes more sporadic, I busy myself with my work and home life, yet my father's shadow always dances on the backdrop of my mind.

Concern about the details of his medical treatment gives way to a powerful, unfulfilled yearning. The truth is, my father has always been a stranger, both from his own shell of privacy and his absence from my childhood. In England, he disappeared at dawn on an early morning train to the hospital where he was training in London and returned home long after my sister and I were in bed. Later, in Canada, he glided away in his sleek white Pontiac to the Manitoba Rehabilitation Hospital and was rarely home in time for dinner. On the tapestry of my childhood memory, there are a few stray knots marking moments of time spent together – such as the day he took me and a friend punting on the river in Cambridge – but these knots are not enough to form a consistent pattern. Even when around, he seemed preoccupied, anxious, aloof, as if he were merely enacting fatherly duties. I coped by acting out the role of a good son: studying hard, excelling at school, trying hard to play sports, but ignoring my deep need for connection and pretending that this was normal, like many boys of that era with absent fathers.

The few moments of connection were, I suspect, often orchestrated by my mother – perhaps in furtive pillow chats when she hissed, "You really must spend more time with your son." Her proddings resulted in awkward episodes such as a surreal "fishing trip" when I was around thirteen. My father had never fished, but one weekend my mother packed me, my father, and some brand-new fishing tackle off to a cabin on a lake in southern Manitoba. Owing to a steady downpour, we never once fished. I lay on my bed reading comic books and swatting mosquitoes, while my father smoked and stared, lost in thought, into the grey drizzle.

I lived with the hope that someday there would be a breakthrough. Some day there would be a moment of playfulness, spontaneity, true affection such as I witness between other fathers and sons and which to this day can bring me to tears.

In 1990, I desperately want my father to stay alive long enough for that breakthrough to happen. Maybe his illness and its sudden thrusting of mortality will be the catalyst for connection. Maybe too, my desperation will be mirrored in his own awakening to the lost opportunities with his son.

I need to act before his cancer gets worse, while he is in the temporary respite provided by the testosterone blocker. I put a plan into action. In the summer, I take my children, by then a girl of twelve and a boy of eight, for a week-long visit to Calgary. I hope this visit will turn into a dual opportunity for connection with me and creation of treasured memories of their grandpa.

When I first see my father, I'm impressed by the improvement in his condition since I last saw him at Christmas. The knotted creases on his forehead from intense pain have loosened. He's walking with ease. From time to time, he smiles. Although his testosterone blocker is supposed to produce minimal feminization, his cheeks have a newfound slightly girlish plumpness and smoothness.

The visit goes well until a picnic at Fish Creek Park, an unspoiled green space wedged between the southern suburbs of the city. It's a beautiful day, with the silver peaks of the Rockies indenting a clear blue sky. The park has an artificial lake fed by the cool, crystal waters of the Bow River, and my children, both avid swimmers, are keen to swim. I deliberately linger at the picnic table to watch my father lead them into the water. This may be the last chance my kids have to play with their grandpa. I want desperately for this to be a happy memory for everyone. My son starts the typical exuberant horseplay of an eight-year-old boy, slapping handfuls of cold water onto my father.

All of a sudden, my father turns on him and gives him a shove, a shove so hard my son falls back and disappears under the surface. When he bobs up, he's crying. He scampers out of the water towards me, face a glistening mask of water, lake mixed with hot tears from the shock of the rough treatment from his grandpa. I pull him into a cold, wet hug.

It's not the first time I've witnessed an eruption of rage from my father. In the spring of 1989, during my training at the Marsden in London, my parents paid us a visit prior to my brother's wedding. As we strolled in a leafy London square, a stray soccer ball almost tripped up my father. Something snapped inside him, and when a boy trotted up to retrieve the ball, my father took an aggressive swipe at his head. Mercifully, he missed. The little boy scooped up the ball and ran away as fast as he could.

There's something about boys that triggers my father. Does he resent their playfulness? Is it a reminder of the lost opportunities for spontaneous fun in his own childhood, spent in the disciplined confines of boarding schools?

My son has inherited my father's dark hair and brown eyes. In fact, he so much resembles my father as a boy that my ailing, semi-delirious grandmother once confused him with her son. At the beach, does my father glimpse a freer, more exuberant version of his younger self? And feel as though he needs to rein him in, the way he always was?

Or does his crankiness have a simple medical explanation? The hormones can cause mood swings and irritability. Maybe too, he's ashamed of the subtle femininization of his body. Small mounds of enlarged breast tissue jiggled over his pecs as he waded into the water.

My son's not physically hurt, but there's a painful gash inside. For the rest of the day, he's wary of my father. I stew in silence, wondering if and how I should respond. Perhaps I should cut my father some slack – the man's got cancer. But if I let it go, it might happen again. And what about my son's respect for a father who doesn't come to his defence?

That evening, after the kids are tucked in bed, my parents and I retire to their basement rec room, festooned with souvenir pennants from the Calgary Olympics and Calgary Stampeders games. As we sip our coffee and make small talk, anger smoulders inside me.

"I didn't like the way you pushed Jonathan today," I blurt.

My father blinks several times, then makes a dismissive wave. "He's too soft."

Soft. The word immediately evokes painful playground taunts from my boyhood in England. "Soft": a boy who is physically weak and overly sensitive. Synonym: "Weed." Both were scalding brands placed on boys with undesirable, repugnant, feminine qualities. Girls are soft; boys are hard, invincible. Weeds like me worked hard to suppress our softness.

"And we all know where he gets that from," pipes up my mother.

"Where?" I say.

"That farm girl. She coddles that boy."

My parents had never approved of my choice of my wife, the daughter of a potato farmer from southwestern Ontario. Conveniently overlooking the facts that the farmer and his wife were highly educated and very engaged in local community affairs, they felt that marriage to a person they sneeringly referred to as "that farm girl" was beneath a doctor's son. Had it not been so fraught, this scenario might be fertile ground for a comic opera featuring a story of young lovers of different social stations whose union is opposed by the groom's parents. It's all played out on a vast potato field where a chorus of rosy-cheeked farm girls confronts a group of handsome white-coated male interns from the city.

The situation was far from comic. At family gatherings, I was ripped between my love for my wife and loyalty to my parents, whose attitude became a permanent throbbing, festering abscess beneath our marriage – an abscess my mother took delight in poking any time an opportunity arose to remind me of my wife's "unsuitability."

On that evening in Calgary, my mother doesn't just poke the abscess, she lances it and releases a torrent of pus. She launches into a tirade with familiar themes: my choice of wife, the wicked influence my in-laws have over me, my faulty child-rearing skills, and my total inadequacy as a parent. I regress to a ten-year-old schoolboy cowering in a corner. I try to defend myself, my wife, her family, my children, but each response fuels her anger until she's a whirling dervish of tears and spittle spinning against the bright pennants of the rec room.

Meanwhile, my father sits silently in his recliner, jaw clenched, eyes darting occasionally at me. He nods like an obedient backbencher listening to a prime-ministerial rant.

I can't bear his silent acquiescence any more. Silence, absence, neglect I've experienced my whole life. Rage rises inside, pushing politeness, respect, compassion aside.

"You old bastard," I blurt.

My cheeks burn. How could I say such a thing to my own father? To a man with cancer?

My mother gyrates close to me, arms flailing. I fear she's going to strike me. "How dare you! Your father's a dying man!" she shrieks. She sobs, then, clutching her housecoat to her neck, turns and stomps off upstairs. My father rises, gives me a hostile glare, and follows.

I collapse into a shrivelled version of myself. The gaudy pennants stare at me in cheery rebuke. *Go, Stamps, Go!* I hear only muffled footsteps and the drone of the air conditioning unit.

My kids and I fly home the next morning. Shivering in the crisp dawn air, we wait for a taxi on the stoop of my parents' house. My mother pads outside in her housecoat and slippers and bids us a coldly formal farewell. My father doesn't come to say goodbye.

At the airport, the gate-number display is blurry. Sensing something's wrong, my daughter, who has inherited my mother's blonde hair and cornflower-blue eyes, tugs my arm and guides the three of us to the correct gate.

Through the aircraft window, I watch the sprawling prairie city recede. As the plane lurches upwards, waves of disappointment, shame, regret, anger, and guilt pass through me. My quest to make connection with my father has ended in utter failure.

"Why are you so surprised?"

Death is in the seat beside me, cradling a glass of scotch in his ivory phalanges.

"Remember Sam."

"Who's Sam?"

"Come on. How could you forget."

~

The morning after our chat where he'd told me he has cancer, Sam goes to the operating room.

Dressed in baggy operating room greens, a paper mask compressing my nose and mouth, I stand beside his unconscious form and watch as Jeff performs the ritual actions of prepping the surgical field in the upper abdomen. A sweet, strangely pleasant perfume drifts from the iodine solution he slathers on the skin. Tiny pools of the golden-brown liquid gather in the creases between Sam's well-defined abdominal muscles; muscles that are about to be incised and forever scarred. To the background rhythm of the chirping of the heart monitor, Jeff clips crisp green drapes around the area, creating a perfectly rectangular window of amber-tinged skin through which the creature in Sam's abdomen is about to be delivered.

An elbow presses into my flank. It's the operating room nurse parking a trolley of gleaming instruments by the bed. "You stand down there." She gives me a slight check with her hip, and I shift towards Sam's feet.

Death hovers in a corner, eyes focused on the surgical field with the intense interest of a spectator just before the opening whistle of a game.

Jeff takes a scalpel from the nurse and examines the point, the shiny tip a reflected silver flame on his glasses. Without hesitation, he presses the blade into the skin just beneath the end of the breast bone. The knife sinks effortlessly, as though slicing through a light, moist cake, and the edges of the incision peel back, revealing the plump white glistening layer of fat beneath. Tiny rivulets of blood trickle from the lips of the wound to the drapes, where they create dark-crimson blotches. Despite its glamourous aura, this business of surgery, of cutting another human being, always strikes me as somehow barbaric and terrifying. I admire Jeff's confidence.

Jeff makes repeated sweeps with the scalpel. Each sweep cuts deeper and deeper through layers of fat, sinew, muscle, and releases the same odour of fresh raw meat I've smelled from a butcher's parcel.

The scalpel shudders as it encounters resistance. Jeff pushes, but the knife won't go deeper. He tosses it onto a tray and inserts a gloved finger in the wound. He wiggles his finger around.

"Holy shit," he says.

Jeff pulls his bloody finger out of the wound. Above her mask, the nurse's eyes rotate to him and her brows gather.

"Can someone call Dr. McCutcheon?" he says.

The nurse shrugs and leaves. Jeff puts his finger back in the wound and wiggles it more energetically.

"Can I ask ... what's wrong?" I pipe up.

He withdraws his finger and points at the wound, now frayed and bleeding from his poking. "Find out for yourself."

I gingerly place my gloved finger inside the incision and probe. The wound is slimy, surprisingly warm, with a pulse at its base. It's the pressure of the aorta filling and collapsing with blood.

"Don't be shy. Go deeper," Jeff says.

The tip of my finger encounters a hard layer.

"What do you feel?"

I make tiny circles with my fingertip. The surface is rough, studded here and there with pebble-like excrescences. I give it a slight push but it doesn't yield. A Kevlar jacket embedded under Sam's skin.

A voice booms over my shoulder.

"You fellows got the stomach out yet?" It's Dr. McCutcheon.

"Uh, I don't think we can get it out, sir," says Jeff.

"What?"

McCutcheon pushes me aside and thrusts a stubby finger into the wound.

"Christ." He withdraws his finger, turns away, and rips off his glove. Drops of blood spatter on the bright green sheets.

"The guy's got fucking *linitis*! Close him up!"

McCutcheon marches out. Jeff starts to sew up the wound.

"*Linitis*? What's that?" I ask timidly.

"*Linitis plastica*," growls Jeff. "Look it up."

"Can I ask why you're not going ahead?"

"Didn't you feel it? Cancer. Plastered all over his abdominal wall. Inoperable. Now stop gawking, hand me those forceps."

Death twirls exultantly.

Sylvia sits in the waiting room outside the operating room, flipping through the pages of a magazine in an uninterested manner. As soon as she sees Jeff and me she jumps up.

"How did it go? Is he okay?"

"He pulled through it great," says Jeff with a fake grin.

"Wonderful. The cancer's gone?"

"Well, it was a tad bigger than expected. We can't remove it right now."

Sylvia's smile vanishes.

"Oh. When?"

"We'll ask the rads team to see him. They'll give him some zaps to shrink it down. Then we'll go back in and take it out."

"Zaps?"

"Radiation. We'll get them to see him tomorrow."

As Jeff and I stroll through the corridor towards the cafeteria, whose location is heralded by salty wafts from the steam tables, I ask Jeff if he really thinks radiation will do any good.

"Nah."

"Oh, then why'd you tell her that?"

"Always gotta give hope, buddy."

"What's going to happen to him?"

"He's toast. Don't look so glum. Win some, lose some. Oh look, the special's lasagna."

Toast? As I pick at my chunk of dried lasagna, the hubbub of the cafeteria fades away as I think about Sam. I can hardly believe what I've heard. Is this fit, friendly man really "toast" – is he going to die? Is there nothing more that can be done?

That night at home I read that *linitis plastica* is a form of stomach cancer in which the cells infiltrate widely through the stomach lining. The medical nickname is "leather-bottle stomach," because the stomach becomes as hard and rigid as a dried-out flask. Sam's leather bottle is stuck to the lining of his abdomen, making surgery impossible. Implacable, unyielding, the creature has refused to surrender itself.

Jeff's prognosis is accurate: nearly all patients with this condition are dead within a few months. It's a rare case that responds so well to radiotherapy or chemotherapy that the cancer can be removed. And even in those rare cases, the cancer often returns.

I close my textbook. When and how will Sam and Sylvia be given this new and even more dreadful news? What new layers of obfuscation will be added to the evasion around his situation that I'd already witnessed?

I didn't need to worry. The next morning Sam is back on the ward. In his room, there's a tall, burly man with a fluffy white beard sitting at his bedside, holding and gently patting one of his hands. A relative? No, the visitor is wearing a white lab coat.

Sam sees me and smiles. I notice a film of tears over his eyes.

"Hi. Looks like I've taken my last flight."

The doctor squeezes and releases Sam's hand.

I recognize the bearded man as Dr. Friar, from the radiotherapy department, whom I'd first met during my summer internship, and who's come to talk to Sam about radiotherapy. I recall how his comforting, Santa-Claus-like presence had overturned my perception of radiation oncologists as geeky and unsympathetic. Here he is again, unafraid to sit at the bedside and hold another man's hand. In my brief medical career, I'd rarely if ever seen such overt gestures of kindness from a physician.

"I've just been filling Sam in on his condition," says Dr. Friar.

I glance nervously at Sam.

"The surgeon said if you give him some radiation, they can remove the cancer later?"

"That's maybe too optimistic. In my experience, stomach cancers don't react well. They're what we call radioresistant."

"What can be done then?" I catch a note of pleading in my voice.

"Radiation will certainly help some of the symptoms. But it's unlikely to make the cancer removable. I've been giving Sam a realistic picture of what his future holds."

Realistic picture. The consonants cut through the fog of obfuscation that had surrounded Sam's situation.

"I'll try the radiation. But my days are numbered," says Sam. "How long do you think I have, doc?"

Dr. Friar's broad brow creases and he takes Sam's hand again. "That's always hard to say. Three to six months, perhaps. In your case, closer to six, because you're in good shape otherwise."

There's silence. Sam gazes out the window.

"Well, I've had better innings than my dad. He didn't make it to fifty."

A wave of sadness passes over me. Dr. Friar stands up, revealing his tall Falstaffian bulk.

"I'll go set up the radiotherapy." Dr. Friar reaches down, gives Sam's hand a final squeeze, then winks at me. "You're in good hands with this lad. Don't worry, we're all here to look after you."

As I watch his immense form trundle away, I think, this is the kind of doctor I want to be. The kind who provides hope and comfort even in a dire situation. I'm still astonished to discover this jewel of humanity in the often brutal and oppressive atmosphere of the hospital.

After a busy day in the OR, I return to visit Sam that evening. Sylvia is sitting by his side. Her eyes brim with tears.

"I still can't believe it. Is it really so bad?" she whimpers, staring at me.

Words elude me. Sam takes her hand.

"Don't worry, love. We'll face this together."

That night, I'm the clinical clerk on duty. Around 10:00 p.m. I'm lying under a coarse blanket on an old-fashioned iron cot in a cramped windowless room in the converted former nurses' residence that serves as sleeping quarters for the on-duty students and residents, thinking of the young women – back then, always women – who wriggled out of their starched uniforms and loosened their hair before collapsing on this same bed after a gruelling day's work a century ago. I'm tired and want to sleep, but the anxiety of being called by one of the wards at any time prevents my alertness from sinking below a light snooze. Just as I start to drift off, the inevitable happens: a voice cackles, witch-like, from the antiquated squawk box at the head of the bed. The nurse summons me to come see Sam; he's in some kind of trouble.

Sam stands by the side of his bed, holding a urinal in his hand, a look of terror on his face.

"Take a look."

He tilts the urinal towards me. It's filled with bright red blood.

"I just peed this."

I tell Sam to rest in bed, trot to the nursing station and call the resident on duty. I'm relieved to reach a friendly female resident, who directs some urgent blood tests.

An hour later, the results are back. They show Sam's developed a condition called disseminated intravascular coagulation (DIC). Tiny blood clots jam the small blood vessels of his body. These clots consume all the proteins normally used for coagulation, resulting in uncontrolled bleeding from other sites. DIC is one of a number of paraneoplastic conditions: complications not caused directly by the cancer but by the presence of the cancer in the body. The invader triggers the release of proteins that in turn provoke the formation of the clots.

I explain this to Sam and tell him the treatment is a transfusion of plasma to replenish the coagulation proteins.

"Transfusion? I'm not sure I want that."

"If we don't do it, you'll just keep bleeding. Maybe even bleed to ..."

"Death? I'm dying anyway. Wouldn't bleeding be a painless way to go?"

Through the window, I glimpse Death's smiling face, nodding in agreement.

Not acting in the face of a problem? My medical training has instilled the instinct to do something, do anything, when faced with a problem, not stand idly by while disease takes a relentless course.

Yet I see his wisdom. He's got advanced cancer. He's going to die. Why treat a secondary condition? Why not allow him to die now? But – isn't withholding treatment helping him commit suicide?

Before I can respond, Sam's belly heaves, and he throws up a gelatinous bolus of congealed blood that looks like a generous helping of liver.

"Oh God," he says, wiping red slime off his chin.

"Why don't we give you one transfusion just to get this in check? You can talk about how far you want to go with Sylvia tomorrow."

"Okay," he nods, and collapses on his pillow.

Overnight, Sam receives a transfusion. By morning, his urine has returned to a healthy golden colour. But the episode has taken its toll: the next morning, for the first time, he looks like a sick person: pale and weak. The illness is accelerating.

Previously, the plan was to send him home to receive his radiotherapy as an outpatient. There is now no way he can be discharged with this unpredictable condition in his body. He needs to be monitored.

"Shit," says Jeff, when I fill him in. "We need that bed for a proper surgical patient."

I call Dr. Friar and inform him of the changes in Sam's condition. A few minutes later, his large figure looms at Sam's bedside.

"Putting you through radiation right now will just make you feel worse."

"I don't want that. And I know it won't do much good."

Dr. Friar smiles, leans, and squeezes Sam's shoulder.

"I'm sure this young lad will do everything possible to keep you comfortable."

"Of course," I say.

Over the next few days, Sam's condition deteriorates. He agrees to another transfusion, but each day he looks sicker and weaker. His sturdy frame withers, and the lustre in his eyes fades. Sylvia remains constantly at his side.

Death sets up vigil in the corridor outside his room.

Late one afternoon, I'm sitting at the nursing station, sipping a coffee and leafing through a pile of notes on a patient who needs to be admitted, when a familiar figure strides up to the desk. For a moment I think Sam's wandered from his room. I look up and find a man of similar sturdy build and black hair.

"Can I speak to someone who's looking after my brother? Sam Park, in 314."

Sheila, a nurse, points her pen at me.

"Hi. I'm the medical student on his team," I say. "How can I help you?"

"Student? I want to talk to someone in charge."

Sheila shrugs. "Dr. McCutcheon is tied up in the OR, honey."

The man beckons me into the corridor.

"I'm his brother, Paul. Flew in from Alberta yesterday. I've brought his mom. The trip did her in. She's resting at the hotel. He told us he has cancer? And he's dying?"

"I'm sorry, yes. Advanced stomach cancer."

"I came by as soon as I got here, but I see *she's* in there."

"You mean his wife?"

"Wife? Girlfriend. What I want to know is, does this hospital impose any restrictions on visitors?"

I point to a sign showing regular visiting hours are from noon to 8:00 p.m.

"Yes. I saw that. I mean, is there a limit on how long one person can visit?"

"I don't know."

"Then find out."

I trot to the nursing station, consult with Sheila, and scurry back.

"She doesn't think so."

"Is it okay for her to hog all his time?"

"I guess, if that's what he wants."

He thrusts out his chest uncomfortably close.

"Look, you need to know something. She's been nothing but trouble for this family. She's the reason Sam and his wife split up."

"Oh. I didn't know that," I say.

"I don't want her spending any more time with him. I want you to restrict her visiting times. Now."

My mouth drops open. I had witnessed only an open, loving relationship between Sam and Sylvia.

Paul's chest shifts even closer. Another step, and I'll be pinned to the wall.

"Uh ... I'll see what I can do."

"Thanks. I'm going back to the hotel to check on Mum. When I come back I expect that woman to be gone."

He strides away and through the exit doors. On his way he peers with disgust into Sam's room.

I pop my head round the door of the office of the head nurse, Ernest, a tall, friendly Black man with small gold hoops glinting on his earlobes. He always has time for medical students. He looks up from his paperwork with a warm smile.

"Hey sweetie. What's up?"

I explain Paul's request.

"Hmmm. I've had no reports of any problems with her. Anyway, like you told him, it's up to the patient. You have any more problems, come fetch me."

I go to Sam's room. He's alone. Sylvia's gone for coffee.

"Good news. Your brother and mom have arrived."

"Oh? Great."

"Your brother just spoke to me. He's worried about you, er, getting tired with so many visitors. We can restrict visiting hours if you like."

"Restrict? Why would I do that?" He looks down at the sheets. "Oh ..., is it about Sylvia? I thought this might happen. Don't mind him. He and Mum never got over my decision to separate from Doreen. I won't go into the details, but it's the best thing I ever did. Sylvia's a wonderful woman."

"I can see that."

"Let anyone who wants to see me, come."

"Including Paul?"

"He's my brother. With what's going on, it may be my last chance."

An hour later Paul appears on the ward. He glances through Sam's door, then makes a beeline for me.

"How come she's still there?"

"It's what he wants."

"What's it got to do with him?"

"I ... uhhh ..."

Ernest sashays out of his office, lowers his glasses, and fixes his eyes on Paul.

"Sir. The patient decides which visitors he gets. Now leave this young man alone so he can get on with his work."

"This is crazy!" says Paul.

"Sam said he wants to see you," I say. "He's pretty sick and ..."

"Not while she's there."

Paul emits an angry snort, stomps away, and bashes the swinging doors open.

Later that same afternoon there's yet another change in Sam's condition. His temperature rises and his pulse quickens. He sits in bed, propped up on pillows, face flushed, hair matted with sweat. He stares at objects on the ceiling.

"Three, four, five, six ..."

"What is it?" asks Sylvia.

"Gremlins. Don't you see them? Gremlins marching up the wall and across the ceiling."

"No, pet, there's no gremlins."

She strokes his forehead. Sam's head drops back on the pillow. He gazes at her.

"Of course, love. There's no gremlins."

Sylvia gives me and Sheila a searching look.

"Poor thing," says Sheila, smoothing the bed covers. "He's delirious. Probably has an infection. The young doctor here will order some antibiotics and something to calm him down."

Sheila leaves, and I swivel to follow her.

"Oh ..." says Sylvia.

I turn back.

"There's something I need to mention. Sam and I talked the other day. He told me he doesn't want to end his life on a machine. He wants to die peacefully. Please don't do anything to keep him alive."

Her words grate against my instinct to be active.

"Uhh ... I'll see what the resident says."

At the nursing station, Jeff sits, munching on a submarine sandwich. I fill him in on the situation.

"Uh-oh. Time for Vitamin H," he says.

Vitamin H is medspeak for Haldol (haloperidol), a strong sedative that's used to quell delirious or unruly patients.

"And what about their request not to do anything? I mean, isn't that ..."

Jeff takes another bite, then flips open Sam's chart and scrawls some orders for Haldol. Then he blocks "DNR" (Do Not Resuscitate) in huge letters across the bottom of the page, shoves the chart to me, and turns back to his sandwich.

I gaze at the stark block letters, smeared with a trail of mayonnaise embedded with particles of lettuce. DNR. Their meaning sinks in. Sam is about to die, and we're not going to stop it.

The Haldol stops the hallucinations, but the infusion of antibiotics does no good. Overnight, Sam's temperature climbs even higher, his pulse becomes erratic, and he becomes drowsy.

Death has caught him in a snare and reels him away, far beyond our reach. Rescue is impossible.

Why am I so terrified? Medical school begins with death – the dissection of cadavers. And on my journey through hospital wards, I'd often glimpsed the drawn curtains concealing the body of a newly dead person. I'd sometimes been asked to participate in the pronouncement of death – but always on patients who were not under my care, who had already died. They were merely anonymous bodies, one step removed from the cadavers in the anatomy laboratory.

Sam's situation was the first time I witnessed Death's cruel dealings up close in a patient who I had got to know as a human being. My education had not prepared me for my feelings of affection for him, forged through witnessing his illness, and resultant sadness and helplessness.

Sylvia doesn't exhibit my helplessness. She remains calm and lovingly focused on Sam's comfort. She offers him water, adjusts his pillows, dabs at his flushed forehead, whispers words of encouragement in his ear, always present, always comforting.

I marvel at how her simple actions soothe him. Simple comforts like this – or Dr. Friar's hand squeezes – are skills not taught in medical school.

As the hours go by, Sam's breathing turns into a harsh croak with a gurgle-like undertone. A trapped, injured sparrow trying desperately to free itself from his windpipe. I'd never heard anything like it before.

"That's the death rattle. Get used to it, honey," whispers Sheila.

At mid-morning Paul appears in the corridor, wheeling an elderly lady with a large sun visor drawn over wispy white hair.

"This is Sam's mother," Paul announces.

"I want to see my son," she says in a regal tone.

"In here," I point to the room.

"Is *she* in there?" she says, hissing *she* as though it's poison.

"Yes."

"Then I'm not going in. Take me back to the hotel."

"I did my best, Mum," Paul says with a hostile glare at me.

"She's got you all around her little finger. Just like she has with Sam. It's all a big show so she can get her hands on his money."

Sheila emerges from the room.

"You'd better go in. Now." she says.

Paul hesitates. Sheila beckons with the firmness of a traffic cop, and he plows the wheelchair into the room. I follow.

Sam is now unconscious, head twisted sideways on the pillow, eyes open but glassy, unseeing. His chest expands and contracts in erratic heaves. For a moment, he appears to stop breathing. Sylvia's arm supports his neck.

Paul parks the wheelchair at one corner of the bed. The old woman tilts her visor back and glares at Sylvia. Her eyes flame with unalloyed hatred.

Paul presses up against one wall, face purple with rage.

No stage director could create a more perfect family tableau of anger and hostility.

Sam moans, then his body deflates. I watch for another breath, but it never comes.

Sylvia cradles his head in her arms. No one moves. No one says anything.

Even faced with death, this family could not heal the cancer within it.

11

The Failed Patient

The rec room spat causes an estrangement from my parents for more than a year. For a few weeks, there's a flurry of letters from my mother, rehashing the incident and her opinions of my ineffective parenting and overprotectiveness of my son. In a ploy typical of her, some of the letters are addressed to my wife. One of them asks for her help in understanding "what is wrong with Charles."

Indeed, what is wrong with me? As I continue my work routine, guilt and confusion eat at me. For the first time in my life, I enter therapy. In a soft recliner in a bright room overlooking the serene Kennebecasis River, I begin the lifelong process of understanding my family origins and the psychic forces that influence me. I learn for the first time the value of simply talking in the presence of a non-judgmental figure.

Late that summer, my family and I move back to Ontario so I can take up a position at a large academic teaching hospital. I'd cut my professional teeth as a radiation oncologist in Saint John, and now it was time to move on to a job with opportunities for teaching and research – as well as an increased salary, an important consideration with two children fast approaching adolescence. I'm sure now awareness of my father's mortality gave added pressure to the desire for a more prestigious position. Time's running out: before you die, I'm going to show you what I'm made of!

The busyness of moving and settling in a new home and job provides a welcome distraction from my father's illness and the conflict with my parents. News from Calgary becomes sparse and predictable: with my father's condition stable, my mother's letters revert to familiar themes of complaints about the weather, gossip about our English relatives, and accounts of various organs' skirmishes with lupus. They enjoy what is to be their last trip to England, and a visit from my brother and his wife with their new baby. I never hear from my father directly. I feel a pinch of hurt by this, but the silence is usual: for as long as I can remember, my mother was their mouthpiece. Anyway, what father would want to reach out to a son that's called him a bastard?

As time goes on, the shadow play of my father's illness on the backdrop of my mind looms larger and more ominous. The oncologist in me knows it's only a matter of time before the hormone therapy wears off. My father's rapidly careening towards the average time – between two and three years – when the hormone-insensitive clones will seize control and his cancer will erupt with greater fury. Maybe, just maybe he'll be one of the lucky ones, one of the few miracle cases I've seen, patients who surpass all statistics and live for many years, their cancers sluggish symbiotic parasites rather than active, rampaging beasts.

It's not to be.

Late one night, just after I've fallen asleep, the insistent ring of the phone breaks the silence of the house.

"Your father's in a coma," my mother croaks at the end of the line.

Yes, my father's cancer is back, back with a vengeance. The cancer has exploded, swelling to a large mass that fills his pelvis and compresses the ureters, leading to a dangerous backup of toxins in the kidneys. As his kidneys fail, poisons accumulate in his blood and flood his brain, and he's lapsed into unconsciousness.

"I'll come tomorrow," I say, replacing the phone.

My wife rouses and blinks.

"What's happened?" she asks.

I tell her the news. She draws me close in a warm embrace.

After she drifts off, I lie wide awake, staring at the mottled reflections of moonlight on the ceiling. I've been expecting this moment ever since the Christmas Eve tidings of two years earlier, but it's still a shock. The hormone treatment has failed. His cancer cells, liberated from hormonal bondage, will now grip my father in a spiralling, downward death waltz. Damn. Why didn't I push harder for total blockade?

Even total blockade is a stopgap that would have given him a few more months at best. A tide of frustration rises in me. I'm face to face with a painful reality: the limitations – I'm tempted to say ineptitude – of my profession in treating metastatic cancer. All the previous decades of research into cancer, and the mountains of cash and intellectual effort they've consumed, seem futile. My profession suddenly feels no better than a gaggle of inept charlatans, hawking vials of unproven remedies to unsuspecting townspeople in a town square.

To be fair, research has produced such approaches as hormone therapy, which has bought time for both prostate and breast cancer patients, and some real permanent cures, especially for childhood cancers, blood cancers, and some rare adult cancers, even when they've spread. Screening programs have helped to improve survival rates for some cancers through early detection of small curable tumours. But for a large proportion of cancer patients, such as my father, cure is not possible. The best some can hope for is for us to "control" the disease for a time using chemicals or hormones; for others, the only hope is relief of symptoms without the use of any specific anticancer agent.

Perhaps my father's current situation will be presented at the local version of the Genitourinary Case Conference. Some pipsqueak oncologist is likely to refer to him as having "failed" hormone therapy. For patients like my father who reach the point at which a treatment no longer controls the disease, oncologists commonly say the patient "failed" a treatment, as if it's somehow the patient's fault. I've often heard colleagues say, "Mrs. X has failed chemotherapy" or "Mr. Y has failed hormones." The truth is, it's the other way around: the treatment failed the patient. Saying the patient failed is yet another of those fuzzy obfuscating scrims found everywhere in oncology. It's deflecting the responsibility for failure away from the doctor and the inadequacies of modern medicine.

Failure is another of those closeted subjects not covered in medical school. Doctors trumpet their successes, rarely their failures. Recent analyses of medical publications have shown the bias towards publishing research showing positive results. A study showing the ineffectiveness of a remedy is unlikely to make the front page of the *New England Journal of Medicine*.

Yet even a cursory look around a hospital shows failure is everywhere: not just failure to cure, but failure to diagnose properly, failure to act swiftly, failure to relieve symptoms, failure to comfort, and – highly relevant in radiation oncology – failure to follow the Hippocratic dictum of "First, do no harm."

~

"What's going on with my leg?"

Tom, a seventy-four-year-old retired firefighter with a craggy face decorated with a bushy seventies' era moustache, leans forward, yanks up the frayed hem of his jeans, and loosens a gauze bandage strapped to his leg.

The bandage drops to his ankle, revealing an oval defect measuring about twelve by eight centimetres on his shin. The defect is so deep I glimpse the ivory surface of bone at its base.

I crouch and examine the wound more closely. The edges are smooth. There's no redness, no lumpiness, no blood, just a clean oval defect. I ask him to flex his ankle. Tendons glide silently over the bone like pistons. I can't resist a surge of wonder. It's like a peep-hole to the hidden machinery of his leg, an animation of a diagram in an anatomy textbook.

I stand up and stare at the wound. I recognize immediately what's happened.

Tom has radiation necrosis. Necrosis, from Greek *nekrotes*, a state of death of tissue, sometimes called mortification. As a result of radiation – *my* radiation – the skin and its underlying tissue in this area has died and sloughed off, leaving this deep hole.

I stare at the wound, momentarily unable to lift my eyes to meet his gaze. A nauseating ripple of guilt sweeps through my chest. My God. He may need amputation.

What do I say? It's my fault. I've inflicted this on him.

I first met Tom a year earlier, when he was referred by a dermatologist for possible radiation for a cancer on his leg. The skin is a vast field exposed to that scorching carcinogen, the sun, and so it's not uncommon for patients to develop multiple cancers over time in different regions. Tom was no exception: scars from previous surgical scrapes, scoops, and snips pitted his face and arms.

But now he had a lesion that could not be dealt with so simply. At that first visit, he drew his pant leg up to reveal a ragged, bloody wound that looked fresh from a shark attack. I'd asked him if he had any history of trauma to the area, and he told me many years ago, he'd been badly burned by an upset kerosene lamp. The area had always been red, but over the previous year a lump formed, a lump which eventually expanded to a crater with a central depression. As the edges of the crater withdrew, they left behind a plain filled with debris: dried pus, coagulated blood, and black clumps of dead cancer cells. Thinking these changes were simply a consequence of the burn, he hadn't done anything until a constant ooze of blood staining his pant leg forced him to his doctor. A biopsy showed the same reptile that clung to Betty's scalp – a squamous cancer. The term for a cancer like this, arising in an area of previously traumatized skin, is Marjolin ulcer, named for the French surgeon Jean-Nicolas Marjolin who first described it in the early nineteenth century.

Tom saw a surgeon, whose opinion was that the area was far too large to be removed with a straightforward operation such as cutting out the tumour and stitching the skin back together. Surgery would involve removal of half the circumference of the skin of Tom's shin, and the defect would have to covered with a skin graft from his buttock. With Tom's history of adult-onset diabetes and heavy smoking, the surgeon was worried the graft would never survive, and Tom would be left with a massive defect on his leg that would expose him to infection, even sepsis. Tom didn't like the sound of this. The surgeon casually mentioned the possibility of amputation of the leg, and that scared Tom into asking if there were any non-surgical options. He was sent to me to consider radiation.

I examined Tom, paying special attention to the areas where his cancer could spread: the lymph nodes in the pocket at the rear of the knee and the groin. I found no enlarged nodes. As I examined him, I noticed the bluish, dusky, slightly swollen appearance of his leg, findings that pointed to a poor blood supply. I lightly pressed my index finger between the tendons of the upper part of Tom's left foot, searching for a pulse. I found none.

He noticed the frown on my face.

"What's wrong, doc?"

"You've got really bad circulation in that leg."

"Yeah. Surgeon already told me. That's why he can't operate. I'm hoping you can clear this bugger up with radiation."

I scratched my cheek and looked sideways at the leg.

"Hmmm ... I'd really rather not do it. With a leg like that, there's a high risk of damage from radiation."

"Holy. No surgery, no radiation. What the hell am I supposed to do?"

"Umm ... well, dressings ... painkillers."

"That's all? Won't the cancer get worse?"

"Umm, well, yes, as time goes on."

"I don't want that," he growled. "I got things I want to do with my life. You gotta do something, doc."

He fixed me with an intense pleading look.

I'm wobbling astride the central pivot of a see-saw with two figures at each end. One is a joyous reveller, Cure; the other, a growling beast, Toxicity. I can't have one without the other: radiation always carries some risk of collateral damage to healthy tissues. Usually, the dose required to cure cancer far exceeds the level at which serious damage is expected, and the see-saw tips towards Cure. In Tom's case, the bad condition of his leg means the risk of side effects is high. If I treat him, I may deliver him into the jaws of Toxicity.

My radiation mentors instilled in me respect, even fear, of toxicity. Once radiation is absorbed by the body, you can't take it out again. Radiation's not like drugs, which can be washed out of the body. Patients don't become radioactive – a common misperception reflected in the frequently asked questions "Will I glow in the dark?" or "Is it safe for my grandkids to sit on my lap?" – but long after the machine is switched off, the effects of deposition of electromagnetic energy in the body remain. In this way, radiotherapy is similar to surgery. Cutting and radiation are both irreversible. Unlike surgery, radiation rarely produces visible scars: its effects are invisible and insidious. Although some healing can occur over time, latent damage often shows up when the tissue is exposed to further trauma such as surgery or infection.

The fear of provoking side effects explains why so much research in radiotherapy is directed at inventing crafty ways of reducing doses to healthy tissues while increasing the dose to cancers. Cancer patients entering a modern radiation department will likely have heard their doctors use acronyms like IMRT (intensity modulated radiation therapy, in which the intensity of the radiation beam is precisely matched to the target volume) or IGRT (image gated radiotherapy, which incorporates imaging of the cancer into the treatment). IGRT originated from the observation that tumours move during treatment. The best example is lung cancer. Owing to normal respiration, lung cancers move, even to the extent that part of the tumour drops out of the radiation beam and healthy lung tissue drops in. I was shocked when I first saw an image of a lung tumour disappearing like the setting sun at the bottom edge of a radiation field as the patient breathed in. The cancer was under-dosed, and the healthy tissue was overdosed. In IGRT, the beam follows the tumour with great precision.

Fear of toxicity explains why radiation oncologists are, by and large, thoughtful, obsessive types, not prone to making sudden, headstrong decisions such as an ER doctor is forced to make. Other specialists become frustrated with the slow, deliberate way we make decisions and the prolonged time it takes to prepare radiation. In radiation, obsession is a necessary art, one encapsulated in a Russian proverb quoted to me by a former patient, a professor of Russian himself frustrated by the length of time it took to arrange his radiation: "Measure the cloth seven times, and cut only once." Because a mistake can have deadly consequences, radiation plans are scrutinized in several quality-control steps before the beam is turned on a patient.

The fear of errors permeates the radiation workroom, creating an unrecognized tension that sometimes bubbles up in irritability. I've been as guilty as any of my colleagues of snapping when I feel anxious about a plan. But often, the tension is dissipated in black humour – such as the day the workroom erupted in laughter because CT images of a patient's innards looked exactly like Porky Pig's face.

This commingling of anxiety, tension, and humour creates a special band of radiation warriors, a camaraderie unique in medicine.

I gazed at Tom's anxious, pleading face.

"Can you give me a minute? I want to pass your case by my colleagues."

Only my fellow warriors would be able to understand my dilemma.

"Sure. But you better bring back some good news." Tom picked up a magazine and slumped in his chair.

I strolled over to the clinic workroom, a cramped, windowless space, and found three of them hunched over computers in small work carrels: Dr. Darwan, a tall, middle-aged man with fading movie-star good looks, Dr. Tsang, a lean, spectacled man with neatly combed silvery-grey hair, and Dr. Ruth, a short, round woman whose wrists glinted with bangles of various shapes. All three pored over radiation maps with the studied focus of air traffic controllers – indeed, they were controllers, trying to avoid collisions between photons and the atoms of healthy tissues.

Dr. Tsang caught sight of me and swivelled.

"Hey, what's up, man?" he said with his customary cheerfulness.

"Got a case I need to discuss."

"Shoot."

I recited the details of Tom's case.

Dr. Darwan's knees began to jig furiously. "Uggh. I wouldn't touch him with a bargepole. The guy needs an amputation," he said, without turning.

"Okay. I wonder ... any role for brachy?" I asked Dr. Ruth.

Brachy is slang for brachytherapy, from the Greek word *brachy*, short. It's radiation treatment from sources at short distance, as opposed to teletherapy, from *tele*, long, beams fired from a distance, as in a linac. It's another manoeuvre for giving a high dose to the cancer while minimizing the dose to deeper, healthy tissues. Dr. Ruth was our department's Queen of Brachytherapy. Her nimble fingers were adept at placing radioactive seeds into awkwardly located body cavities or tumours.

She had a technique for skin cancer that involved thin hollow tubes loaded with radioactive wires placed over the face of the tumour. It's the modern equivalent of the "Elastoplast mould" I witnessed as a student. The behind-the-scenes preparation steps and calculations were complicated, but it was easier for patients because they could come for only one or two visits.

She turned and peered at me over the top of her half-moon reading glasses, fastened to her neck by a thin gold string adorned with tiny glimmering pendants.

"Thickness?" she asked.

I showed her the CT images of Tom's leg on her computer. The cancer showed as a deep bite on the front of his shin. Dr. Tsang leaned in and peered at the image between our shoulders.

Dr. Ruth tutted and shook her head.

"Wow. That's a whopper," she said.

"Amputate!" muttered Dr. Darwan.

"Too thick for brachy. I'd never be able to get any dose down to the base. Sorry."

She adjusted her sparkly chain and turned back to her computer.

Two strikes. I turned to Dr. Tsang. The gleam in his eyes told me the sight of Tom's cancer had aroused his inner warrior.

"Yeah! I'd treat him."

"Lawsuit! Lawsuit!" barked Dr. Darwan.

Dr. Tsang rolled his eyes and leaned in to me.

"But I'd go slow," he whispered.

By "going slow," he meant reducing the daily dose. There's a correlation between daily fraction size and toxicity – the higher the fraction, the greater the risk of permanent damage. If I can keep the daily dose low, I may be able to reduce the risk of damage to Tom's skin.

"I had a patient like that a few months ago. She's done well."

"Hmm. Not a bad idea. Thanks."

As I slowly walked back to the clinic, I thought, yes, I can go slow with Tom. But for that to work, I'll have to extend his treatment to eight weeks. He's already told me he's keen to get up north for the hunting season.

Outside the door of his examining room, another thought stopped me. If I lessen the daily dose and spread his treatment over many weeks, I may reduce his chance of cure. During radiation, tumours undergo a phenomenon called repopulation, in which cancer cells replenish. The dose of radiation has to be strong enough to counter this. If I back off too much, the cancer may never react and disappear.

I pushed the door open and plunked myself on the stool opposite Tom. The gaping red wound on his leg stared back.

Tom looked up from his mag.

"Uh-oh. Don't tell me it's bad news."

"I'm still not sure," I said.

He tossed the mag aside and sat up straight.

"Look, doc. Why don't you tell me what you're thinking and let me make up my own mind?"

Yes. That old hubris again. I hadn't really given Tom enough information for him to assess his own situation and make an informed decision.

There was nothing wrong with inviting Tom to climb on the see-saw with me so we can survey the risks together.

I explained to Tom that there might be a way to treat him, but I couldn't guarantee it would cure him or spare him side effects.

"There's no such thing as a free lunch," he said with a smile. "Let's do it."

His smile dissolves when I tell him it's going to take eight weeks of daily visits.

"Holy. Eight? I've already booked the hunting lodge."

"It's really the only way I can treat you safely."

His moustache twitched and he frowned.

"Okay, doc. Guess I'll change my plans."

Tom proceeded through a planning process similar to Betty's. The therapists fashioned a rigid sleeve to keep his leg immobile during treatment, I drew my magic circle around the tumour, and he had a CT scan.

Radiation patients always question why they need another CT when they may just have had one ordered by another doctor. It's because the scanners in the radiation department are specially equipped to transform the images into data useful for plotting treatment – in particular, data about the density of different tissues, which affects the absorption of radiation. For skin cancer patients, the CT also serves to assess the depth of the tumour below the skin surface, something which cannot be assessed with the naked eye.

Once I know the depth of the cancer, I can select an appropriate intensity of radiation. The linacs produce beams of different intensity. As the intensity goes up, the beam penetrates deeper.

I peered at the images of Tom's cancer through the window of my computer playhouse. Unlike Betty's, this *squame* looked more like the outcome of a reptile attack than the reptile itself. There was a large, deep defect with ragged edges from the creature's frenzied gnawing. This appearance is characteristic of some skin cancers and gives rise to the term "rodent ulcer," like a rat has nibbled away at the flesh.

I was about to measure the depth of the cancer with the electronic ruler when something caught my eye. I looked closer. Thin black tendrils of cancer reaching inward and brushing against the front of the big bone of the lower leg, the tibia. I was quite sure they weren't present on his earlier scan.

My God. Just like Matthew's, Tom's cancer had grown. To encompass it all, I would have to use an intensity that saturates the entire thickness of the soft tissue of his leg right down to the bone. This would increase his risk of side effects, and maybe even injure the bone and lead to complications such as infection or spontaneous fracture. I've had patients whose previously irradiated hips or arms suddenly snapped from thinning caused by radiation.

I leaned back in my chair. Its springs gently rocked me back and forth. My eyes met the figure of Death in the Saliger engraving.

"Quit acting the hero."

"Shut up. This isn't like Matthew. I know I can cure this guy's cancer. I'm just worried about what I'll do to his leg."

There was a soft rap on the door.

"Come in," I said, and Dr. Tsang entered, coffee mug in hand.

Death froze in his usual posture in the image.

"Hey, man. Burning the midnight oil?" he said. Then, after glancing at my screen, "Oh, you're working on *him*."

"Take a look at this," I said, pointing to the new wisps of cancer brushing against the bone. "I don't know what to do."

Dr. Tsang took a sip from his mug, leaned in, and studied the image. The gleam in his eye told me his inner warrior had stirred again.

"You told the guy about the risks? You're going slow?"

"Yes," I said.

"Then just do it, man."

I heard something like a groan from the area of the Saliger engraving.

I grabbed my mouse and clicked. A menu fluttered down from the flies behind the proscenium. I clicked again beside the highest intensity on the menu. Then a final click sent a command to begin the chain of activity that will ultimately unleash a fury of radiation on the leg. As my palm relaxed from the mouse, I recalled the dusky appearance and weak pulse of Tom's leg, and a wave of anxiety passed through the pit of my stomach.

Because of the go-slow approach, Tom sailed through radiation with no side effects other than mild reddening of the skin around the cancer. He was curious why he also noticed some redness and itchiness on his calf, opposite to where the radiation was directed.

"Some of the radiation is exiting through the skin," I explained. "It'll clear up once the treatment's over."

By the third week, his cancer was withering. By the end of treatment, it was almost gone. Tom was delighted and made plans to catch the last few days of hunting season.

"You like moose meat?"

I mustered a weak smile. "Uh, no, I'll take a pass. Thanks anyway and good luck."

Over the next few months, healthy skin reoccupied the site of the malevolent *squame*. Tom proudly showed off his healed leg to his buddies.

But, a sinister process was occurring beneath the superficial healing. Radiation has caused intense inflammation in the tissues deep beneath the skin. As if girding themselves against further trauma, these tissues began to knit a steely armour of fibrosis, a thick matrix of scar tissue that squeezed and suffocated his already thin, weak blood vessels. Starved of oxygen, the tissue in this area started to die. As it did so, a sinkhole appeared on the surface of the skin, a sinkhole that eventually collapsed and opened to become the deep crater visible at Tom's most recent visit to me.

"What's going on?" Tom repeats. My silence has made his tone more insistent.

I lift my gaze to his face.

"It's from the radiation."

His eyebrows lift in surprise, then gather together in a frown. For a moment, I fear retribution: Dr. Darwan's cry of "lawsuit" rings in my ears. But then, his expression softens to benign puzzlement.

"Oh – so this is what you meant by damage?"

"Yes."

"Jeez. I never thought it would be this bad."

"I'm sorry."

I force a cheery smile. "The good news is there's no sign of cancer."

He gazes down at the hole in his leg.

"So, now I just have to live with this? Or can something be done?"

No plastic surgeon will operate on a wound like this. Besides, it would just give them more fodder for their already sceptical attitude towards radiation.

"Well, wounds like this sometimes heal on their own."

With a wound this size, the chance of healing is low, but I feel compelled to say something optimistic.

Tom smiles. "Great!"

I explain as long as the area is kept clean and free of infection, there's a chance that over time the healthy skin at the edge will slowly creep in and cover the defect. I remind him of the importance of good nutrition, especially adequate protein intake, for healing.

Kim, the nurse working alongside me that day, gives Tom instructions for cleansing and dressing the wound, and I arrange to see him again in a month.

After Tom leaves, I slump in the workroom, consumed by regret and guilt. I've delivered Tom into the jaws of Toxicity. I've transgressed the Hippocratic dictum "First, do no harm." I should have listened to Dr. Darwan's warning. I shouldn't have given in to my warrior instinct. Now look what I've done.

The small consolation is that Tom's wound – damage to soft tissue on a limb – is not life-threatening. If similar damage occurred in another part of the body – the bowel, the lung, or, worst of all, the brain – the effects might be devastating. The most serious complication for Tom might be infection, which could turn into sepsis, but infection can be avoided if the wound is kept clean.

With any luck, Tom's wound will heal on its own. I sigh and reach for the next patient's file.

At his next visit, Tom unravels the bandage. I measure the wound. It's the same size.

"Hmmm. It hasn't changed."

His lips twist in exasperation.

"Honest, doc, I've been doing everything you told me. Eating right, cleaning it three times a day. Don't believe me, talk to my girlfriend, she's been helping me look after it. We're both getting fed up. There's got to be something else that can be done."

I reach deep into my mental sleeve of tricks.

"There's always hyperbaric oxygen."

"What's that?"

"They put you in a chamber and pump the air pressure up. The extra pressure pushes oxygen deep into the tissue."

"Oh, yeah, I heard about that. I got a navy pal who got it for the bends. Does it work for this kind of problem?"

"Sometimes."

Because the radiation damage has been caused partly by oxygen starvation, hyperbaric oxygen can indeed help to heal wounds like his.

"Cool. I heard some NFL players use it for injuries. Yeah, they call it a miracle sleeping bag. Let's give it a shot."

I refer Tom to a local hyperbaric clinic and arrange to see him again in a couple of months.

Over coffee, I tell Dr. Tsang what's happened.

"Sorry, man," he says, placing his hand on my arm. "Shit happens. But you did warn him about it. And you got rid of the cancer. He's still got his leg."

Tom receives a series of hyperbaric oxygen treatments. Two months later, new lines of weariness etch his face.

I stare at his wound in disbelief. It hasn't changed. Everyone else I've sent for hyperbaric oxygen has had at least some healing. The oval excavation stares back: cold and defiant, an affront to my knowledge. Tom may have to live with this wound for the rest of his life.

"Well, let's carry on for a few more sessions," I say.

Tom reluctantly agrees to have a few more hyperbaric treatments. I continue to see him at monthly intervals. Before each visit, I hope today will be the day when the wound shows signs of healing. But at each visit his increasingly disgruntled look tells me nothing has happened.

"I'm not going back to that chamber. It's a goddamn waste of time."

There's really nothing to do other than monitor him. As the months go by, the hope of healing fades. I start to dread my encounters with him – just as he must dread seeing me.

Then, slowly, almost imperceptibly at first, the reason for the lack of healing becomes apparent. At one visit, I notice a red lump at one corner of the wound.

I hear a faint voice from somewhere in my memory. Yes, it's one of my radiation mentors telling me to never, ever, assume a wound after radiation is just from the radiation. Always consider another, grimmer possibility: persistent cancer.

"Hmm," I say, running my finger over the raised area. "That's new."

"What is it?" Tom gazes at the lump in puzzlement.

"I'm going to send you back to your dermatologist to find out. I don't want to scare you, but sometimes the failure of a wound to heal is due to more cancer."

Tom jerks like he's been electrocuted. "Holy shit."

"I think we need to rule it out."

A biopsy from an area with poor blood supply carries a risk of causing the tissue to break down further and making the wound worse. But I need to find out what's going on. So, I send Tom back to his dermatologist with a request to take some samples.

A couple of weeks later, I'm sitting in my office late one afternoon, signing off a pile of lab reports on my desk.

Tom's biopsy report is among them. I unfold it with anticipation and dread.

It's as I thought. The biopsies show active, thriving cancer cells strewn within the tight whorls of the fibrotic tissue. Through the past months, hidden deep in his leg, cancer cells were wrestling with healthy skin cells, holding them back from forming a healing layer.

Death swivels towards me with a triumphant grin.

I avoid his look by dropping my gaze to the pile of papers on my desk. My body slumps, crushed by an overwhelming sense of failure. My "go slow" approach was too timid. It didn't hammer the cancer hard enough. But it was enough to cause irreparable damage.

I've both damaged and failed to cure Tom.

Then, there's a sudden feeling of relief. I finally have the answer to why his wound didn't heal, why the weeks of antiseptic measures and hyperbaric treatments didn't work. I can tell Tom the truth.

I sit up, pick up the phone, and leave a voice message for Kim to squeeze Tom in to see me the next day and also organize an appointment with an orthopaedic surgeon for him.

Months later, I spot Tom in the lobby of the hospital. He's sitting in a wheelchair by the entrance. His empty pant leg droops over the stump of his left leg.

I lower my gaze and swivel away.

"Hey, doc. Don't be a stranger," he calls.

I turn back, muster a smile, and move towards him.

"Hi. How are you doing?"

"Just in for some physio."

I take a big breath. "I'm really sorry for what you went through."

He gazes deep into my eyes.

"Don't be sorry," he says, with a smile. "You did your best. Cancer's a tough critter. Harder to take down than a bull moose."

"But your ..." I say, pointing to the stump.

"Ah, that old peg. Remember, the first surgeon I saw told me I might have to have it off. Thanks to you, we got another year together."

He gives me a wink, shoves the wheelchair forward, and jerks its front wheels into a wheelie.

12

The Shunned Patient

In the days after Sam's aborted operation, during which his cancer was found to be inoperable and thus incurable, I notice how, during morning rounds, the surgical team stops visiting him. Jeff shoves the cart laden with patient files past the open door of Sam's room like a flight attendant hurrying the drinks cart past a drunken passenger. He acknowledges Sam's presence with only an occasional brief glance at the lonely, bedridden figure within. The only contact is through the nurse when she requests a new order for a sedative or painkiller. It's like Sam has some deadly infectious disease Jeff doesn't want to risk catching.

The disease is failure, wafting from Sam's room like a toxic miasma. Jeff has lost interest in a patient who is a reminder of the impotence and futility of surgery in some situations. I sense too that his training hasn't given him the skills to interact with a dying patient. He knows how to explain the intricacies of surgery but doesn't know how to talk to someone who's dying.

Radiation oncologists are particularly familiar with shunning, one symptom of doctors' inability to deal with failure. Among all the patients sent to us, there's a large collection with relapsed cancer for whom previous treatments, surgery, or chemotherapy have failed. Many have received multiple courses – typically referred to as "first-, second-, and third-line" – of drug cocktails that have rendered them into those bald, pale, near cadaveric beings familiar from media depictions of cancer patients; others have been subjected to increasingly disfiguring surgery as surgeons try to chop or scrape recalcitrant tumours away. We Rad Oncs are the last stop on the line before it veers to its dead end. These patients are sent to us with often plaintive requests: "Anything you can do for this fellow?" frequently accompanied by false encouragement: "Don't worry – Dr. Hayter will fix you up with a bit of radiation."

When I ask such patients if the referring doctor has plans to see them again, the usual answer is "No." The surgeon or medical oncologist has handed – some might say dumped – the responsibility for the patient's care on me. In my experience, it's a rare surgeon who continues to see cancer patients after the failure of surgery. I become the oncologist of reference, the guide in the darkest part of the forest. On the few occasions when I've asked the referring doctor to continue to follow a patient, the typical response is, "I've nothing more to offer." True in the technical sense, but it leaves patients bewildered and lost. Requests for assistance from the family doctor are often met with resistance from both patients and their families, who don't want to sever their connection with the cancer centre, and also from family doctors themselves, who generally consider the complexities of cancer to be outside their scope. In recent decades, specialists in palliative care have filled some of the gaps in care that occur for patients with relapsed cancer, but patients tend to confuse palliative care with terminal care and are resistant to referral. My palliative care colleagues prefer to be involved as early as possible.

Sometimes in my clinic, as I survey the waiting room crowded with patients who have been failed by surgery or chemotherapy, it's as if I'm standing on a seashore, helping survivors of a shipwreck struggle to gain an insecure footing on shore.

Lori's left breast is missing. In its place, a fuchsia-coloured blotch sweeps from her armpit to her breastbone. From the other side of the examining room, the shape is oddly familiar. Yes, it's as though she has a map of Australia glued to her chest. The northern tip of Queensland juts up into her armpit, the shores of Western Australia lap against her breastbone, and a craggy island, Tasmania, floats below the left lower border.

"Can I take a closer look?" She nods, and lifts her gown higher as if drawing a curtain on a stage set. I roll my stool forward. Up close, the features of this new landscape come into crisp focus. Its raised edges form cliffs overlooking wide, sweeping bays of healthy pink skin. Small violaceous outcroppings, some of which have crater-like pockets at the tips, stud the interior. Tiny pools of blood and pus glimmer in the base of the larger craters. The stink of rotting flesh hovers over the landscape, a geothermal field of recurrent cancer.

The show ended, she drops the gown. I roll back. I scold myself for making such an improper geographical comparison. Such unbidden whimsical associations arise frequently in my work: they are the mind's mechanism of distancing me from the true horror of the disease.

"The surgeon said you could fix this. I'm counting on you, doc."

The note of pleading in her voice catches me off guard. I look up at her face. My inferior position lower than her perch on the examining couch renders me small and vulnerable, and for a moment my professional mask drops, and we gaze at each other not as patient and doctor, but as two human beings. I see a vibrant woman, only fifty-four, with clear blue eyes like my mother's and a scalp of brassy stubble, the burned-off field of recent chemotherapy. Flecks of flour on her wrists betray her work as a professional baker. I envision her in some pre-dawn kitchen, happily warbling country and western songs as she pummels recalcitrant loaves. Even though I've known her for only a few minutes, I already like her for her directness and the way she made gentle fun of my wide outdated tie. "Holy. Is that a bib, doc?"

I wish I could "fix" her.

I stand up, turn my back, peel off my latex gloves, and wipe the sticky film of sweat from my palms. I take a deep breath, reposition my mask, command my cheek muscles to lift the edges of my lips to a smile, and turn back.

"Sure, we can try some radiation," I say, with the casual tone of a chef suggesting an untried spice in a recipe. I hope she hasn't caught the tightness in my voice that gives away my misgivings.

"So, will it cure me?" asks Lori.

Uh-oh. She's uttered the dreaded C-word, as loaded for oncologists as the other C-word, cancer, is for patients.

I stare hard at the blood pressure apparatus behind her shoulder on the wall.

Most people's understanding of cure is zap! – total obliteration of cancer. Immediate opportunity to live the expected lifespan of a healthy person of the same age. But it's not so easy. Cancer is sneaky and unpredictable – and often slow. For many cancer types, it takes many years of check-ups to ensure the disease is completely gone. Even then, the survival curves – the plot of survival versus time – can continue to dip like an amusement park ride with no buffer at the end of a slope. I once saw an elderly woman who developed a recurrence on the skin thirty years after her mastectomy for breast cancer. Faced with this uncertainty, oncologists often resort to vague terms such as "local control" instead of "cure" – that is, eradication of the tumour in one area rather than complete, whole-body cure.

For Lori, it's possible my radiation will achieve local control of the disease on her chest. But permanent cure? I'm not sure. Her condition, chest-wall recurrence of breast cancer after mastectomy, is not in itself life-threatening, but is often the harbinger of metastases elsewhere in the body – to liver, lungs, or brain – that will be fatal. Lori's lucky: right now, unlike many women in her situation, her scans have shown no sign of cancer elsewhere in her body. So, yes, there is a small chance of cure, a small chance of riding down the survival curve until she glides to a halt on a flat strip of track. But right now, today, she's still too high up the slope to know when or whether its curve will end.

I look back at her face, open and alive with curiosity. The drawstrings in my cheeks pull my lips upwards again.

"Ummm ... we'll have to see how it goes. We'll do our best."

It was Dr. Friar, the radiation oncologist of Falstaffian proportions whom I first met at Sam's bedside and who later became my teacher, who introduced me to the metaphoric shorthand of oncology. "See here, a good example of *peau d'orange*," he'd intone, thick fingertip stroking the characteristic pockmarks of the skin of the breast caused by choking of the underlying lymph channels by cancer. Or "Look at those *cannonballs*!": showers of metastases, round white meteors hurtling through the night sky of a patient's lungs on an X-ray. Or "Notice the *winking owl*," a radiological anomaly formed by the lopsided collapse of a cancerous vertebra. Skin tumours are "strawberries" and "cherries"; "cauliflowers" sprout in the throat or rectum. I learned that these metaphors are a handy, compact shorthand, more precise and vivid than the scientific term, useful for communication between oncologists. A colleague knows exactly what I mean when I say I've got a patient with a "big cauliflower on the tongue." Dr. Friar taught me the term *carcinoma en cuirasse* to refer to Lori's condition.

A cuirass, a jacket of steel protecting the torso, is familiar to anyone who's wandered the halls of European armouries. Henry VIII's massive pigeon-breasted, gleaming cuirass still evokes awe at the Tower of London. For a time in the Victorian period, there was a vogue for bodices shaped like cuirasses, cinching the waist and thrusting the breasts towards the chin.

Carcinoma en cuirasse is shorthand for recurrence of breast cancer on the chest wall after removal of the breast. A few cells, possibly dripped from the edge of a scalpel fresh from slicing cancer, form an invisible colony where they multiply, grow, and eventually send offspring into surrounding territory. These offspring swarm through the subterranean channels of the skin – ever multiplying, ever pushing, ever crowding – until they form a rigid girdle of cancer. In their feverish quest to conquer, these marauders can outstrip the supply chain of blood, leaving oxygen-starved compatriots to die in festering pits or charnel heaps of tumour – the pebbles and craters of Lori's chest.

Doctors and patients alike frequently ignore or misdiagnose carcinoma en cuirasse in its early stages. Encouraged by the illusion that removal of the whole breast guarantees cure, they brush off early symptoms with "It's just a rash" or "It's only a pimple" or "It's just scarring from surgery." Then, one day, out of the blue something sinister happens: one of the pimples erupts, sputtering blood, or the rash starts to expand and swell, like one of Lori's yeasty loaves. Even in the presence of these symptoms, patients, abetted by their doctors, often persist with useless topical salves. Finally, in the face of unremitting pain or bleeding, a doctor takes a sample of the skin and submits it to a pathologist for microscopic examination. One glance in the microscope is enough to divine the patient's future.

As a man, I can only summon faint imaginings of the terror of a woman who goes through both amputation of her breast and recurrence of cancer despite surgery. Spread of cancer to the brain, spine, or liver is frightening, but these manifestations are invisible, their presence manifest only on scans or through symptoms such as pain, nausea, or headache. A woman with brain metastases from breast cancer can gaze into a mirror and perhaps fleetingly forget the horror hiding in her skull. But for a woman with carcinoma en cuirasse, there is no hiding, no ignoring, no forgetting.

Does Lori stand behind the locked door of her bedroom, robe parted, gazing at the stippled, erratic smear of cancer on her chest? No wiping or scrubbing will remove this stain. What does she feel? Fear, self-loathing, shame, confusion, helplessness? Will my partner ever want to hold me again? I went through mastectomy for *this* to happen?

And her surgeon? After its development by Johns Hopkins surgeon William Halsted in the 1890s, the radical mastectomy became the supreme symbol of surgical power over cancer. Spurred on by mastectomy, surgeons devised similarly radical operations for cancers throughout the body. Cancer was thought to spread centrifugally from its point of origin, so the removal of all tissue adjacent to the cancer would guarantee cure. No organ – bowel, bladder, stomach, uterus, oesophagus, throat – was immune to this dogma. The consequences of heroic surgery – disfigurement or loss of normal bowel, bladder, or sexual function – were considered small prices to pay for cure. Amputation became the standard recourse for penile cancer.

Carcinoma en cuirasse shows how easily one tiny, recalcitrant cancer cell can overturn this dogma. Removal of the whole breast and adjacent tissues, even the pectoral muscle, does not guarantee cure. Rarely, it can be detected early enough to be removed, but usually by the time it's diagnosed the area of recurrence is so big no further surgery is possible. It becomes a visible, palpable ugly rebuke to surgical power. In its presence, surgeons become helpless, impotent spectators.

Face to face with failure, little wonder that surgeons often banish such women from their clinics. They shunt them off, down the backstairs to the dim corridors of the basement radiation department, to see me, then strike them from their books. Along the way there may be a brief unproductive detour to the chemotherapy department for a trial of ineffective drugs.

A few days after her first visit, I meet Lori again in the Simulator. When I arrive, the staff have already set her up in the treatment position. Swathed in a flimsy blue gown, she's lying on the treatment table on her right side, arms raised, head resting on her right elbow, left arm draped over her forehead, with a pillow tucked under her right flank, thrusting the cancerous part of her chest up. Immobile, she's a victim of Vesuvius, terror petrified.

It's my job once again to delineate the "target volume" so the radiotherapy staff know where to direct the deadly beams. Magic marker in one hand, I draw back the sheet covering the tumour. One of the therapists wheels a spotlight into position. Under its bright glare, the cancerous bloom is bigger, redder, and angrier than I remember.

I survey the area, pondering where to put my lines. A beam with finite edges will deliver the radiation, but the disease in front of me is potentially infinite. Beyond the edge of the visible tumour, invisible fugitive cells already burrow under apparently healthy skin. There's no test to reveal these outliers. To my naked eye, it's impossible to know exactly where cancer ends and healthy skin begins, to know with absolute certainty where to place my marks. Because of this uncertainty, I draw my lines three or four centimetres from the edge of visible tumour and thus leave a DMZ of healthy pink skin between the tumour and the edge of the radiation beam. But even this wide margin may not be enough. It will take only a few cells beyond my marks for the radiation to fail to control the disease and doom Lori to yet another outbreak.

Marker poised, I stand at Lori's side, momentarily daunted and anxious. The therapists stare at me with barely concealed looks of frustration at the doctor's indecision.

Lori's face twists towards me from under her left armpit. She's caught my frown, the hovering of the marker in mid-air.

"What's wrong, doc? You are going ahead, aren't you?"

"Sure," I say, and advance the black tip of the marker towards her chest.

In my uncertainty, it's some consolation to know the problem of carcinoma en cuirasse has perplexed, even exasperated, many generations of radiation doctors before me. One of the earliest photographs from the history of radiotherapy, circa 1900, shows a woman with a cluster of tumour nodules sprouting from a mastectomy wound. Like the figure in Saliger's engraving, her naked figure reclines before the glass bulb of a primitive X-ray apparatus. She waits patiently to absorb the rays shortly to sputter from its tiny filament.

Later, the problem vexed Dr. Gordon Richards, the mustachioed, dictatorial head of radiotherapy at Toronto General Hospital, one of the early twentieth-century leaders who set the previously careless practice of radiotherapy on a new scientific footing. In response to the dual challenge of the widespread infiltration of cancer in the skin and the application of a flat beam of radiation to a curved surface, he came up with a novel device: the "radium jacket."

Throughout my career, I'd heard radiation oncologists who were senior to me mention this fabled device and always wondered what it looked like and how it worked.

One day, I descend to the dusty, windowless stacks of the medical library and locate the fat volume of the journal *Radiology* from 1934 containing Richards's article, "The Treatment of Chest-Wall Secondaries in Breast Carcinoma: A Preliminary Report of a New Radium Technic."

There it is: on the first page, a greyscale image of a headless female torso wearing what looks like an old-fashioned cork life jacket such as might have been used on the *Titanic*. Its outer face is covered with row upon row of shiny needles sewn to the fabric. According to the text, the jacket held one hundred needles, each with a cavity filled with three milligrams of radium – tiny nuclear reactors generating invisible gamma rays. The rays emitted from the needles coalesced to form an envelope of radiation moulded to the torso of each patient. As I gaze at the photograph, my face flushes with excitement at discovery of this vivid historical image – or maybe it's a sympathetic response to the radiation?

Radium was discovered by Marie and Pierre Curie in 1898. It's a naturally occurring substance, refined at great labour and expense from ochre-coloured uranium ore scoured from the earth of Western Africa or the Northwest Territories of Canada. Its atoms are in a state of constant but sleepy disintegration: it takes 1600 years to dwindle to half of its original amount. As they disintegrate, they discard energy in the form of gamma rays.

It was observations of the damaging effects of radium that gave birth to the field of radiotherapy. If radium damaged healthy tissues, then why not diseased ones as well? Spurred on by enthusiastic reports of its seemingly magical powers, by the early years of the twentieth century doctors were figuring out how to apply radium to every crevice of the human body – using flat applicators, tubes, or, as in the case of the radium jacket, needles.

Within those needles, the disintegration continues relentlessly, day and night, week after week, year by year. There's no on/off switch: the only way of containing the volatile emissions is to lock the radium away in a lead-lined safe. As I gaze at the images, I can't help wondering: whose nimble fingers sewed a hundred needles on the jacket? Did Dr. Richards take the felt vest home to his wife? I see them in the comfort of their living room, sitting across from each other in front of a blazing fire, he poring over a medical journal, she carefully stitching the needles, a dim ethereal glow reflected on her face. Perhaps she drops one, and there's a frantic search on the carpet for the precious needle – in the 1930s, gram for gram, worth more than gold.

More likely, the sewer was a minion with scant if any awareness of the unseen danger. Richards alludes to a dressmaker who fitted the jacket – was it she, or possibly he, who also sewed the needles in place? It seems unlikely that a hospital had a full-time dressmaker, so from where was she recruited? From the ranks of immigrant seamstresses in the sweatshops of Spadina Avenue? Someone who barely spoke English, who could little comprehend the danger of her work – just as dangerous, if not more so, than the work of the famous radium dial painters of New Jersey, whose jaws disintegrated from repeatedly licking the tips of radioactive brushes. Even the most dexterous seamstress could not avoid handling the needles, and thus develop a mysterious rash, or blistering – even autoamputation – of fingers. Or, as the radiation leached into the body, were the effects more insidious, bringing her into the sisterhood of female radiation martyrs such as Marie Curie, whose lifelong exposure to radiation eventually poisoned her marrow.

And what of the other women – those who wore the jackets? No names or faces appear in the article. The women are reduced to a panel of images of female torsos lined up like marble effigies on a museum shelf. Richards says each woman wore her life jacket for four days. Strapped in their jackets, alone in lead-lined cubicles, anxious, waiting, wondering: what did they feel? Likely nothing but a mild itch while the jacket was in place. Perhaps some were relieved the treatment seemed so easy.

Like the disintegration of radium itself, the effect of the gamma rays is slow and insidious. Relief dissolves when, after a few days, crimson patches appear in the treated area, patches that coalesce until the entire area is bright stop-sign red. Next, the entire surface begins to bubble, blister, and weep murky, straw-coloured fluid. Then, the surface layer of dead skin and cancer cells sloughs, revealing a sheath of glistening raw salmon. The nurses apply dressings and salves of zinc oxide and castor oil, but the searing pain is relentless. The women become modern versions of Medea's victim Glauce, whose flesh peeled off from a poisoned robe.

At this point, some women develop fever and delirium and must be admitted to hospital. At long last, spring arrives: tiny pink shoots of new skin break through the surface, shoots that spread and blossom exuberantly until the entire surface is a smooth flat field of rosy, healthy skin.

The radium jacket healed cancer for some women. But exactly how many? And for how long? Were any permanently cured? Richards's article has no statistical summary of the results. He merely concludes with a time-honoured cliché of medical non-commitment, one that likely conceals his own misgivings: "The results are promising."

Eighty years later, when Lori comes to see me, the radium jacket has long been relegated to the junkyard of radiation gadgets deemed "promising" but too complicated, expensive, and dangerous to introduce into widespread practice. I'll treat Lori with a more sophisticated version of the apparatus used by my predecessor from 1900. Instead of X-rays, we'll use a beam of electrons, shaped to fit my inked outlines, shot from the mouth of a linear accelerator. The electrons plummet beneath the surface of the skin, where they scatter and careen, and eventually settle into a fatal waltz with the delicate spirals of DNA in the nuclei of the cancer cells. There's a big advantage of electrons over other particles: their weak penetration. They deplete all their energy within a few centimetres and thus don't damage the delicate lacework of the underlying lung.

Lori receives twenty-five doses of electrons, five days a week, for five weeks. Once a week, after her appointment on the machine, she's booked to see me in my review clinic for a check on how she's doing. At these visits, in a common gesture of radiation patients, she brings a gift for me and the staff. The first week, it's a paper bag stuffed with buttery oatmeal-raisin cookies fresh from her oven; the second, a tray of lemon cupcakes crowned with bright yellow icing and sparkling golden sprinkles.

Like the women who wore the radium jackets, at first Lori feels nothing other than a slight tingling in the treated area – the result of blood rushing in to defend an area of assault.

"This is a piece of cake!" she chortles, as she slides the cupcakes on the reception counter.

In the third week, the appearance of her chest changes. There are signs the treatment is working: the raised edges at the margin of the cancer smooth out, some of the tiny pools of pus dry up, and the nodules collapse. At the same time, the healthy DMZ of skin around the cancer begins to dry and redden into an arid, sun-baked desert. The electrons are non-partisan and pair up indiscriminately with DNA in both the cancer and healthy skin cells.

The fourth week, Lori lugs a tray of plump, sticky cinnamon buns. The odour of cinnamon wafts through the radiation department, luring curious radiation therapists from their consoles to my desk. The tray quickly empties as they stuff chunks of gooey sweetness into their mouths.

This week, I can tell something's wrong with Lori. She seems less energetic, and her blue eyes have lost their lustre.

I discover the reason when I examine her. A massive branding iron has stamped a fiery imprint of the same shape as the radiation beam on the chest. Here and there, blisters bubble from the surface as if the radiation has summoned hidden magma from beneath. As my fingers probe, Lori recoils.

"Owwwww. Please no."

My hand jerks back. Her cry reminds me that, even though the reaction of the tissue is expected and is a routine part of radiation that I've seen many times before, for Lori it's a new and terrifying experience.

"I'm sorry," I say.

At this point, many patients get angry: "If I'd known radiation was going to be like this, I'd never have gone through with it."

Anticipating a similar outburst from Lori, I ask, "Would you like a break?"

Her eyes expand in puzzlement.

"Hell, why would I want that?"

"A few days off would give your skin time to recover. The pain will improve."

"Yeah, and give the cancer a break too?"

"Maybe at least you should consider taking some time off work. All that movement irritates the skin."

"Nah. Work takes my mind off this."

"At least let me give you some painkillers."

"No, doc. I can take it. Let's keep going."

I persuade her to take a prescription anyway, just in case, and Ivy gives her instructions for cleansing the area.

At the end of the final week, she plunks an enormous cardboard box on the counter. It contains a massive cake covered in snowy white icing. She's swirled *Thank You My Lovely Radiation Peeps* in pink icing across the top. Pink rosettes dot the corners. As she waves goodbye to the radiation staff, tears glisten in her eyes.

After she leaves, someone finds a scalpel, and I carve the cake into cubes. I distribute the morsels of sweet sponge to the staff on improvised plates of paper towel. For a moment, the sounds of satisfied grunts and the greedy slurps of icing licked off fingers permeate in the radiation department.

A month later, Lori returns to see me for a checkup. She bounces in to the examining room. Those friendly eyes gleam again.

Before I even ask, she hoists the side of her gown like a royal unveiling a plaque.

"Take a look, doc!"

Her chest, a few weeks ago trapped in a cuirass of cancer, and more recently set ablaze by the radiation, is completely healed. A faint bronze outline corresponding to the shape of the radiation area is the only sign of her treatment. Like the sun, the electrons have coaxed the sleepy melatonin-producing cells – responsible for pigmenting the skin – to life.

"Wow," I say.

"Yeah, wow," she says. "It was sure hell but it was worth it. The pain's gone, and guess what? I can wear a bra again. I've even dug out my left falsie."

I slip on my latex gloves and perform a routine check. My fingertips slide over the treated area. It's flat, smooth, pristine.

Yes, wow indeed. As with Betty, a result like this reignites the wonder I felt as a resident when I first witnessed the seemingly magical effects of radiation.

My fingertips glide over the skin. A few centimetres out from the DMZ, they bump up against something hard nestling under the skin. I probe deeper. Yes, a tiny pebble just under the surface. And a centimetre away, another.

I know immediately what they are. Two colonies of fugitive cells. Colonies outside the bounds of my carefully placed marks.

Damn. *Damn*. The radiation has worked, but only in the area it was directed.

Failure.

I pull my hand away. I drop my gaze to the floor tiles. My mask of cheerfulness loosens and begins to slip. Deep inside, despair, frustration, and inadequacy churn their rotors.

I want one of the floor tiles to open up like a trapdoor to a perfect world of no defeat, no failure – the fantasy Wonderland of medical school.

"Is everything okay?" says Lori.

I swivel away and stamp the pedal of the garbage can. Its jaw snaps open, and I toss my gloves inside. I stare into the tangled debris within. What went wrong? Maybe my marks were too close. Maybe these nodules were there before, and I missed them.

What do I say? What do I tell her? How can I destroy this moment of joy – perhaps one of her last?

I stand, take a big breath, and reposition the loosened mask. I turn and look into her beautiful eyes. They gleam with anticipation.

No. Not today.

"Yes, so far, so good. I'd like to keep a close eye. Can you come back in a week?"

13
The Stoic Patient

A few hours after the call about my father's coma, I'm on board the 6:00 a.m. flight to Calgary. I've packed a dark suit suitable for a funeral in my bag.

As the flight attendant performs his bored pantomime of safety instructions, my thoughts are already out west. What have my father and mother been told? Do they understand the gravity of his situation? Do they know he has entered the terminal phase of his illness? And *how* have they been told – with honesty or evasion, gentleness or bluntness?

The disclosure of cancer relapse vies with a cancer diagnosis as the most difficult conversation in oncology. If I had to choose, I'd say relapse is more difficult. At diagnosis, there's hope, maybe even promise of cure. Relapse erodes hope and is an admission of failure. Like a sea monster emerging from the deep, uncertainty pokes its snout above the previously calm seas: now that treatment has failed, what comes next? At diagnosis, the oncologist and patient were strangers, but by the moment of relapse, they've built a relationship, often over years, based on trust and even mutual affection. Relapse undermines the relationship: How could you let this happen to me? Why didn't you do better? Why didn't you give me other options? Relapse brings disappointment, guilt, and confusion, and there's a strong temptation to draw those well-worn scrims of obfuscation, evasion, and procrastination.

In my training and practice, I'd often turned to my well-thumbed copy of Dr. Robert Buckman's 1988 classic *I Don't Know What to Say* for guidance. Buckman was a pioneer in medical communication skills, particularly, as the title suggests, around difficult subjects such as cancer relapse and death. His book is in essence a collection of scripts for breaking bad news and contains tips for breaking the impasse of communication that frequently occurs around fraught subjects. He suggests the use of open-ended questions such as "What do you understand is going on right now?" to pry open the conversation with a patient or family.

I'd often found Buckman's script book helpful in my own encounters with patients. I hope my father's doctors in Calgary have used similarly gentle, non-threatening techniques.

Even with all the rehearsal in the world, breaking bad news remains a difficult task.

~

Every Wednesday morning, my trajectory to work takes me north on Highway 427 past a landscape of squat industrial buildings, west past an array of vivid red control beacons of the airport, and finally north again into a leafy, quiet suburb settled by many South Asian immigrants. As I approach the hospital, I spot bearded men in turbans and women in bright saris out for early morning walks in the sun.

On this particular hot, steamy August Wednesday, my forward momentum slows and finally stops as I pull up behind a vast herd of immobile vehicles. I peer through my windscreen and glimpse the reflections of white and red flashes of emergency vehicles on the concrete walls of the expressway. Another accident. It's 8.40 a.m., and my clinic at the local hospital starts in twenty minutes. I'm going to be late – again. There's nothing to do but sit here, crank up the radio, and listen to morning talk-show prattle. The summer sun beating on the roof slowly turns the car into an oven. To hell with global warming. I crank up the A/C. Nobody wants to see a doctor with a shirt glued to his skin by sweat.

I'm headed to a peripheral clinic, where radiation oncologists assess patients in a hospital without its own radiation treatment facilities. If radiation is required, patients must travel to the cancer centre.

Weekly trips to such outposts have been part of my work since I started my career. In my first job, in New Brunswick, the provincial radiation centre was in the gritty port town of Saint John, and my territory was the staid capital city, Fredericton. I got up at dawn for an early morning drive along the serene Saint John River to the Fredericton hospital, a squat Lego-like building. In my trunk I hauled fat suitcases stuffed with patient files resembling the cases of a travelling salesman. Indeed, there was a sales aspect to my work, for I often had to convince both reluctant patients and their sceptical doctors of the need for radiation. By the time I left the hospital, mentally numb from the day's encounters, darkness had descended on the river. Once I rounded a curve and encountered two enormous moose, black figures motionless in the gloom, and at the last second managed to direct the nose of my car between the rump of one and the nose of the other.

On one level, peripheral clinics are a pain, since they involve both tiring commutes and interruption of the workflow at the base cancer centre. Little wonder that Rad Oncs try to dodge them when responsibilities are being handed out at staff meetings. But they serve an important need for patients. Radiation machines are expensive to install and operate, and so in most countries of the world radiotherapy is highly centralized. Centralization has been one of the chief principles of the planning of oncology services ever since the notion of special clinics for cancer emerged in the early twentieth century. Back then, many experts felt the concentration of equipment and expertise in cancer clinics would lead to better care for patients, as well as enhanced research opportunities. Dr. Claudius Regaud, chief planner of France's anticancer system in the 1920s, summarized the doctrine of centralization – and its marginalization of patient needs – when he said, "There is no important reason for placing special establishments for anti-cancer treatment in close proximity to patients." In Ontario, Canada, the commission charged with setting up a cancer program in the 1930s followed Regaud's advice and recommended the establishment of only three radiotherapy centres in the cities with medical schools. (Only in the United States, where cancer care remained rooted in a private, commercial model, did radiation centres proliferate in small communities.)

What about the patients who lived at a distance from radiotherapy centres? It's not difficult to imagine the challenges for patients due to the zealous emphasis on centralization in such vast jurisdictions as Ontario. If you lived in a big city with radiation facilities, it was easy to get radiation treatment, but if you lived in a small, remote community, it was almost impossible. How would you get there? Where would you stay? As early as 1939, statistics from the Ontario Department of Health showed that the further a cancer patient lived from a cancer clinic, the less likely he or she was to be seen there. Geographic inequities in access to care continued and resulted in anomalies such as a higher proportion of women living in outlying areas receiving mastectomy rather than breast-conserving therapy (lumpectomy followed by radiation) for breast cancer. A woman loses her breast simply because she doesn't have easy access to a radiation facility.

The peripheral clinic was one solution. If the radiation couldn't be brought close to the patient, then send the radiation specialists to the patients. They could assess patients in their local hospitals, decide if radiation therapy is appropriate, and arrange treatment at the cancer centre. This idea became so entrenched that on every morning of every week somewhere, someplace, a radiation oncologist climbs into his or her car to make the trek to a peripheral clinic.

Besides patient care, there's a grander educational purpose. In remote communities, there's often a lack of knowledge of radiation therapy. I've sometimes been shocked by how little is known. Once, in the course of setting up a peripheral clinic in a small-town hospital, I was asked if I would be willing to see my patients in a room with four stretchers, normally used to prepare and apply casts for fractures. I was supposed to rotate among four patients in the same room, carrying on fraught and supposedly confidential discussions about cancer with each patient within earshot of the other three. I guessed the suggested arrangements were based on the familiar myth that I'm just a technician. Confronted with such attitudes, I sometimes feel like I've stepped back in time to my grandfather's era in colonial India to become a British tutor whose mission is to educate the locals in the unfamiliar customs and uses of radiation.

It's always a busy day. As I dart from room to room, working my way through a list of pre-booked patients, local doctors often interrupt with queries about their own patients, and sometimes request assessments of extra patients, usually inpatients, the sickest of the sick, those who are breathless, bleeding, or in pain from cancer. They add to the workload, but I never resent being asked to see sick inpatients, because otherwise they'd have to endure a bumpy, swaying ambulance ride to the cancer centre for a consultation, sometimes just to be told I don't think radiation will help.

I don't want to paint too bleak a picture of these hectic clinics. They are a "day away," a welcome break from the routine at the base hospital, and a chance to interact with doctors, nurses, and clerical workers who are often genuinely curious and eager to learn about my field. And the atmosphere in a small-town hospital is usually warmer and more convivial than in the sprawling healthcare "complexes" where radiation oncologists are usually stationed.

On this hot Wednesday morning, the traffic north still creeps along. Up ahead, I see the emergency vehicles blocking several lanes, narrowing the highway like plaque in a coronary artery. It's now past nine. I can hear the muttered curses of the patients in the crammed waiting room ahead. At least we're moving slowly, and my car rolls into a band of shade under an overpass.

I glance at the printout on the passenger seat of the names of patients I'm to see today. Some of the names are unfamiliar: new patients, coming for their first assessment. Others are well known: patients coming for follow-up visits after their treatment. The names evoke mental pictures of their faces and situations.

One name, Christie, stands out. I've known her for almost a year. She's a vibrant, relentlessly upbeat fifty-five-year-old divorcee and real estate agent who's got an aggressive form of lung.cancer, small-cell carcinoma – so called because under the microscope the cancer consists of sheets of tiny indigo-blue cells. This subtype of lung cancer used to be called oat cell carcinoma because of the resemblance of the cells to grains of oats. Their small size belies their behaviour, for these dainty blue cells form one of the most aggressive of human cancers. These malevolent oats coalesce to form great blue-black blobs of cancerous porridge that quickly plug blood vessels and travel to other parts of the body.

When Christie's cancer was first discovered, it was confined to her left lung. For patients such as her, there is the possibility of cure with several months of chemotherapy and radiation to the chest. Because of the potential rapid spread of small-cell carcinoma, treatment always starts with chemotherapy, which subdues the primary tumour and saturates the rest of the body to prevent any stray invisible cells from taking root. Radiation is, to use yet another food metaphor, "sandwiched" between chemotherapy doses.

Because the body is already weakened from chemo, the side effects from radiation are often worse than if radiation was being used on its own. Shortly towards the end of her course of radiation, Christie developed severe oesophagitis – painful inflammation in her oesophagus that made it impossible to swallow anything other than thin soups. Like Lori, she accepted this hardship with cheerfulness. "No pain, no gain!" she said brightly to me one morning, as she lay propped up on pillows in a hospital bed, looking thin and wan from the lack of proper nutrition. After a week, her swallowing returned to normal, and she continued with several more doses of chemotherapy.

Often, the most aggressive cancers, such as small-cell carcinoma, respond most rapidly to treatment. Like quickly drooping peonies, their exuberant growth makes them somehow weaker, more fragile. After the dual assault of chemotherapy and radiation, the mass in Christie's left lung disappeared, and she returned to part-time work as a real estate agent, specializing in vacation properties in the verdant hills and valleys north of the city.

Even after aggressive treatment, those little blue cells can lurk in the dark corners of the body. The brain is a favourite site of refuge, a so-called sanctuary site for cancer, because it has a thick membranous covering that renders it impermeable to chemotherapy drugs. In a healthy person, the blood-brain barrier stops toxins reaching the brain, but in cancer patients, it keeps a potentially life-saving toxin out. In the deep convolutions of the brain, cancer cells can hide, regroup, and gather strength for a fierce counter-attack. It's therefore routine practice to offer patients such as Christie prophylactic cranial irradiation (PCI) to prevent cancer from showing up in the brain. Blasting radiation through a seemingly healthy brain may sound barbaric, but research has proven that it not only reduces the risk of brain metastases but also improves survival from the cancer. The dose of radiation is low, less than half of what is used to treat a primary brain tumour. Because of the sensitivity of the hair follicles to radiation – a phenomenon put to novel use in the early days of radiation, when women sought X-ray treatment for facial epilation – the most visible side effect is thinning of hair. It generally grows back after a few months.

The chief concern of PCI is that for a few patients, radiation can cause a form of mild dementia. My patient and I stand again on the pivot of that teeter-totter, balancing benefit with harm. The risk of side effects must be weighed against the risk of the return of cancer in the brain, which can cause more devastating symptoms than a brain fog. And once cancer returns in the brain, it is no longer curable.

I've discussed PCI with Christie on two previous visits. On both occasions, we've discussed its benefits and risks, but she's always been reluctant. I pointed out her young age and previous good health make her risk of side effects low, but she's afraid of the radiation turning her into a "vegetable." She's still exhausted from her chemotherapy and also doesn't like the inconvenience of having to travel once again to the cancer centre, with its grim reminders of her earlier ordeal, for the preparation and delivery of the two-week course of treatment.

"I thought I was done with that place!"

She lives in a small town several kilometres north of the city, so the return trips for treatments will occupy a whole day and thus interfere with her work. She's concluded both discussions with a friendly but firm "Not right now. I'll think it over." However, she agreed to be monitored with regular CT scans of the brain to make sure there's no sign of a return of cancer. Today she's coming back to get the report of her most recent scan. As I think of her situation, I hope it will be all clear.

There's a roar of revving engines punctuated by honks. The clot on the highway dissolves, and the traffic surges ahead. I sit up, step on the gas pedal, and zoom northward.

Twenty minutes later, I pull into the hospital parking lot and weave through its alleys in search of an empty spot. At length I spot the rear end of an SUV backing hesitantly out of a space, and I quickly slide the front of my car past its nose. The driver, a tiny elderly woman in a sari, gives me a hostile frown over the rim of her steering wheel.

Dazed from the hot, long, stop-and-start drive, I stumble from the car and tuck my crumpled shirt into my pants. I desperately need a coffee, but the line-up's too long at the shop in the lobby. I wedge my way into an elevator filled with visitors and staff, and ride up to the sixth-floor oncology clinic. This is one of the hospitals still not yet brave enough to call it a cancer clinic.

The elevator door slides open, and I encounter Yush, a short, stocky, grey-haired man wearing the pale blue smock of a hospital volunteer. He's pushing a cart laden with a carafe of coffee, empty cups, and a basket of candies.

"Morning, doc!" he says brightly.

I've known Yush ever since I gave radiation to his wife for metastatic breast cancer. I've never forgotten the patient, calm way he translated my information into Mandarin for his wife, who'd never learned to speak English since their arrival in Canada from China. Since her death, he's been devoted to volunteer work in the oncology clinic, dispensing coffee and cheer to patients in the waiting room.

He notices my covetous gaze at the carafe.

"Go ahead. Help yourself."

As I fill a cup, he picks a candy from a basket, gives me a friendly wink, and slides it into my pocket. "Have a good day, doc."

Coffee in hand, I head towards the clinic area. The examining rooms are already full with patients waiting to see me. Through the open doors, I glimpse both relieved smiles of welcome or hostile frowns of impatience.

I spot Christie in the first room. She's wearing a big floppy straw hat with a pair of oversized sunglasses perched on the brim, a bright blouse with a flowery print, and stylish canary-yellow culottes. She belongs on the deck of a cruise ship instead of in a cancer clinic. She gives me a friendly smile and, with a melodramatic wave, yells "Finally!" I remember the reason for her appointment. I feel a slight flutter of anxiety. Will her scan be okay?

I enter the cramped workroom at the end of the corridor, plunk myself in front of the computer, and gulp a mouthful of coffee. As the caffeine percolates to my brain, I locate the report of Christie's scan in the computer files.

I don't need the coffee to perk me up. The report is enough to jolt me wide awake.

"There are new findings of innumerable supra- and infra-tentorial enhancing masses, compatible with brain metastases."

I sit up straight and stare at the screen in disbelief. It can't be. Maybe I have the wrong patient. No, the name at the top of the report is correct.

There must be a mistake. I open the program showing the actual images on which the report is based.

There's no mistake. There they are: clusters of irregular grey globules, floating in the dark convolutions of her brain, distorting its normal contours. A shower of grenades waiting to explode inside her skull.

I stare at the images, letting their meaning sink in. The cancer has returned in her brain. Those cells that had lain dormant for many months have erupted with renewed energy. Her cancer is back, it's no longer curable, and she'll die within a few months. Some palliative radiation may buy her some time, but she's going to die.

I have to explain all of this to her. Right now, she's sitting in the room, contentedly leafing through a glossy real estate magazine. I'm about to pronounce a death sentence on this vibrant person. Will I find the right words? How will she react?

As I draw the coffee cup to my lips, I notice it's shaking slightly. My heart thumps in my chest. There's a film of sweat on my palms. Come on, get a grip, you're a doctor, it's your job to give patients their test results, even if the results are bad. You've done this many times before. You know the Buckman script, something like "I'm afraid I have bad news ..."

Why is this still so goddamn difficult?

If truth be told, it's because I like Christie. Yes, I like her as a person. Since the early days of my career, I've always had patients I've liked – not because they're compliant with my recommendations, but just because they're nice people: friendly, open, easy to get along with.

Doctors are not supposed to get attached to their patients. They are supposed to cultivate something called "clinical detachment." I'm not exactly sure where this concept originates: there's no course in medical school called Detachment 101. I'm not referring to romantic or sexual attachments, which are, of course, wrong. I'm speaking of an emotional bond born from accompanying another human being on an arduous journey through sickness and often towards death. It's ironic that in radiation oncology, widely perceived as a purely technical specialty, such bonds can be very strong. They are forged at the very first visit, when

patients are seen at a vulnerable moment in their lives, just after a cancer diagnosis, and strengthened during a multi-week course of radiation,
when patients are seen at least once weekly. Over a several-week course
of radiation, both patient and doctor alike loosen their masks to reveal
something of the humans underneath. It's hard to ignore the nuances of
an individual patient's personality and see them only as cases.

Such attachments are not necessarily positive. Patients, like family
members, are not chosen and can be just as annoying as the clan gathered around the Thanksgiving dinner table. At any time, there's always
a small group of patients in my practice that I dislike. I came to dislike
Justice McNichol, for example, because of his bullying tactics. There
may be medical compatibility between the disease and the expert, but
not always between the two humans involved. Mistrust and anger can
be as much a part of the clinical encounter as friendliness and compassion. In these cases, the polite, reserved professional mask remains
firmly attached.

Some doctors reading this will bristle. They believe emotions have no
place in the examining rooms of the nation. They're worried emotions
might distort clinical judgment: if you like a patient too much, you might
give that patient more time, extra tests, or preference for treatment slots.
If you dislike a patient, you might skimp on your assessment. I think
there's a middle ground where doctors have to be vigilant against distor-
tions of decision-making but at the same time mindful of their humanity.
Human connection is an integral component of medical practice. It's
another teeter-totter, one that pivots between professional persona and
human being.

So, yes, I admit my fondness for Christie. Like Higgins in My Fair Lady,
"I've grown accustomed to her face," accustomed to her indestructible
cheeriness, directness, and independence. Like many of my patients, over
the course of a few months she's turned from a stranger into something
approaching a friend.

I don't want to tell this vibrant person her cancer has returned in the most terrifying of places: the brain. I don't want to tell her the meaning: she's dying. I don't want her to die. I'm also scared of her anger, maybe even rejection. You put me through months of chemo and radiation, only for *this*? Was it all for nothing? I want to see someone else!

Before going to her room, I glance again at the sinister grey globules in her brain.

There's a familiar musty odour. It's Death. He's standing next to me, eying the images with a smile.

"Pretty, aren't they?"

"Damn. I should have pushed her harder on PCI," I say through gritted teeth.

"You are a soft touch compared to some of your colleagues."

He's right. Some colleagues take a hard line and tell patients PCI is mandatory. They sometimes minimize the side effects of PCI to sell it.

Death's bony finger jabs my shoulder.

"You really should consider coming over to my team."

I take a final gulp of coffee, stand up, and tuck Christie's file under my arm.

"There's nothing to do but tell her the truth."

Death blocks the door.

"Why don't you make it easier for yourself? Use one of those dodges like 'Your brain scan shows a few abnormalities.' 'There are some spots in the brain.' 'Your scan doesn't look right.' Or just mark time. Put it off. Order another scan – 'just to be sure.'"

"No. I'm not going to pussyfoot around. She deserves better."

I shove past Death into the corridor.

"My, my," he says. "Growing balls. Well, mind if I tag along?"

"Okay. But only if you wait outside."

I head towards Christie's room. A figure tracks towards me. It's Dr. Hussein, a short, middle-aged woman with black hair twisted into a tight bun, round wire spectacles, and a regal air. She's one of the local medical oncologists. She fixes me with a stern, professorial look. I know what she wants.

"Hi. Was looking for you. Can you squeeze in a couple more patients?"

My clinic is already fully booked, but I can't say no. Both of the patients she wants me to see are sick inpatients. Making them travel to the cancer centre for assessment is unkind. I say, "Of course," and ask her to give their information to the nurse so I can locate them later. She seems irritated at my asking her to perform a clerical task but nonetheless gives me a polite smile and glides towards the desk.

Christie's daughter Paula, a thirty-something replica of her mother, has arrived, and now sits with her parent in the room. Her face is clouded with concern that contrasts with her mother's sunniness.

I muster a cheery tone as I close the door behind me. "How are you doing?" I ask.

"Great!" says Christie.

She hands me a small glossy brochure.

"Mom!" says Paula.

"Thought you might be interested."

The brochure's a real estate listing for a cottage on a lake north of the city. I scan the pretty pictures of the cosy living room with a picture window overlooking the water.

"Nice, but, whew, pricey," I say.

"Come on, you're a doctor, you're loaded!"

I smile and hand the paper back. She grins back at me.

"I'm feeling great, so I guess my scans are all clear?"

I hate moments like this: my patient says she's feeling great, but I know her body is not. It's hard to believe that behind that radiant smile and beneath that straw hat, her skull is chock-full of cancer.

I stare at her. I've forgotten my lines.

She notices my hesitation.

"They are okay, aren't they?"

I sit and look straight into her eyes. The script returns: "I'm afraid it's bad news."

Paula puts her arm around Christie and draws her closer. "Oh no," she whispers.

Christie stares at me with wide-eyed curiosity. "Yes?"

I forget to breath, and my next sentence comes out all dry and squeaky.

"The scan shows the cancer has come back in the brain."

Paula squeezes her mother. My gaze drops to the floor tiles. I'd never noticed its myriad haphazard scuff marks, etchings from the heels of thousands of anxious patients who've sat in Christie's seat before.

There's a long pause. Paula whimpers quietly. I wait, gazed dropped, girding myself against an outburst of grief or anger. But it doesn't come.

"Okay. Okay. So how long do I have to live?" Christie's words are quiet, measured.

"Mom!"

"Stop. I want to know."

I lift my gaze to Christie's face. Her expression is open, curious.

"You really want to know?"

"Of course."

"Well, most patients in this situation live less than a year."

Through the door, I hear the swish of Death's robes as he pirouettes in victory.

Paula gasps. "Oh my God." Tears stream down her face. I hand her a box of tissues. Christie pulls her closer.

"It's okay, dear. Time to start planning my celebration of life. You know how I love parties."

"Mom, please!"

"I'm really sorry," I say.

"Don't be sorry," says Christie. "It's not your fault. I've been expecting this. All along I thought my cancer wasn't really curable."

Is her calm reaction a result of one of the spots in the frontal lobes causing blunting of emotional responses? I carry out a brief neurological examination, and everything is normal. None of the tumours is exerting enough pressure to cause any symptoms.

"Something has to be done. We can't just let her die," says Paula.

"I can give you some radiation," I say.

Christie gives a melodramatic shudder. "We've talked about that before. No way."

"This time is different. Before it was preventive; now there are spots of cancer to treat."

"What will that do for her?" asks Paula.

"It will likely give you a few more months."

"How many treatments?"

"Just five." With the conversation turning to the practicalities of radiation, I suddenly feel on firmer ground.

"A few months. Let's go for it," says Paula.

"No, sweetie. It's not worth it. The trips, the baldness, loss of memory."

"You've got to do something," says Paula.

"Yes," says Christie. "I do. Start planning that celebration of life."

"Mom!"

Christie squeezes her daughter's hand. "Calm down, dear. Everything's going to be all right. I've told you all along I'm not scared of dying."

Death emits a disappointed squeal.

Christie rises and pulls her daughter to her feet. "Let's go, dear. I'm sure the doctor has other patients to see."

"I'll send a report to your family doctor. If there's anything I can do, please call me."

"Thank you, doctor." She reaches into her bag and fishes out the glossy brochure, and thrusts it into my hand. Her eyes meet my gaze with gentle compassion.

"You have such a hard job. I'm sure you need a place to unwind."

Christie pulls Paula into the corridor. Death makes a low, courtly bow, then follows as they walk towards the elevator.

As I watch them wait at the elevator entrance, the dying mother supporting her trembling, weeping daughter, I feel sad. I'll never see her again. Then admiration cuts through the sadness. If somebody told me I'm dying, I'm sure I wouldn't take it so well.

I go back to the workroom, sit, and flip through the brochure. Green trees, rolling hills, shimmering lakes. Maybe she's right – maybe I do need a country retreat.

Yush pops his head around the door.

"You okay, doc?"

"Fine," I mumble.

He offers me the candy basket. "Have another."

He leaves. I slowly unwrap the candy and pop it in my mouth. For a moment I savour the rich, sweet, caramelly taste. I reach for the next patient's file.

14

The Interfering Child II

Halfway through the journey, the plane passes over Winnipeg, where my family landed in Canada thirty years before. As I gaze down at the sprawling city, once the gateway to Western Canada for hundreds of thousands of immigrants, I remember the cheerful optimism of my parents as they began a new life in a country similar to and yet very different from their homeland of England.

For my father, that life is drawing to a close. Left untreated, kidney failure can kill a person in a few days. I sip tepid airline coffee and urge the lumbering jet to accelerate so I can get there before he dies.

I'm reminded of another teaching of a radiation oncology mentor. He and I stood at the bedside of an emaciated elderly woman with an abdominal tumour so protuberant she looked to be in advanced pregnancy. Like my father's, her cancer obstructed the ureters and caused her kidneys to fail. As the toxins percolated to her brain, she drifted in and out of consciousness. Wrapped in his dark shroud, Death waited in a corner of the room.

Her renal failure could be treated with drainage tubes or dialysis. The professor quietly explained to the patient and her family that kidney failure would allow her to have a painless, comfortable death, and prevent weeks of future suffering from her advanced, progressing cancer. He told them it was their decision, but his recommendation was no medical intervention other than measures to ensure comfort, such as painkillers.

There's an old term for this approach: "masterful inactivity," when, in the face of recurrent cancer, with all treatments exhausted, doing nothing, allowing "nature to take its course" is best. It's accepting the presence of Death and inviting him to step forward and gather the patient into his arms. It's a passive approach, quite different from medically assisted death, which involves the active administration of a deadly poison.

I hope my father's doctors are wise enough to offer masterful inactivity to him, and I hope he considers it. I don't want my father kept alive just to endure more suffering.

But it's not my decision to make. As long as he is mentally competent, it's up to my father to make decisions about the extent of his treatment. Because of the estrangement, I don't know whether my parents have had discussions with his doctors about his wishes around life-threatening medical events such as renal failure, or if he's recorded his decision in what would now be called an "advance directive." How far does my father want to go? Does he want to be kept alive at all costs? A bigger question lurks: Is he ready to die?

Even when patients have clearly expressed their wishes, it's easy for things to get thrown off track.

~

It's a sunny Sunday morning in August. Coffee in hand, I stroll onto the inpatient ward to make rounds on the patients of our department. Making rounds is the morning ritual of checking each patient, responding to nurses' questions or concerns, writing notes in the chart, and adding new orders. In the old days, the doctor making rounds would be attended by the chief nurse; these days, I do it on my own.

It's not a pleasant duty, for radiation inpatients are the sickest of the sick, and the environment is unpleasant. The ward is in an old part of the hospital, built in the 1970s, with oversized fading tangerine stripes on the walls, the relic of some designer's notion of cheeriness. The nursing station, with a bank of computer monitors, racks of patient charts, and counters strewn with reports, is the hub. From this command post, spokes of dimly lit corridors, crammed with wheelchairs, IV poles, and linen carts, radiate to patient rooms. The air holds a bouquet of chemical-floral scents from disinfectants and soaps with rich undertones of feces, urine, and vomit.

Radiation inpatients fall into one of three groups: those with side effects of radiation so bad they have to be hospitalized, those bedridden from serious complications of metastatic cancer such as severe pain or spinal cord compression, and terminally ill patients receiving comfort measures as their lives draw to a close. The hospital has a palliative care unit, but its beds are always in short supply. As a result, many dying cancer patients remain on our ward.

As I enter this dingy, sad place to begin my rounds, the thought that the morning visit from the doctor may be one of the few bright spots in the patients' day energizes me.

As soon as he sees me, Jason, a young freckle-faced nurse, leaps from his seat behind the nursing station.

"There you are," he says, with a tone of admonishment at my tardy arrival. In the absence of urgent calls, I had lingered at home to savour coffee and croissants on the deck.

"I need you to see 477 right away."

"Uhhh ... Does 477 have a name?" I say, batting back his tone.

Nurses are not immune to the reductionism endemic in healthcare. They reflexively identify patients by room number.

Jason locates the chart of Room 477 on the rack and heaves it across the counter. It's a massive tome, cover worn and ragged, bloated from the reports stuffed inside. 477 has been here a long time.

Pinned to the cover is a notice with a wide red border and "DNR" in big bold letters stamped in the middle. DNR = Do Not Resuscitate.

Warning: if this patient's heart or lungs fail, he or she is not to be revived.

I flip through the pages. "Oh yes. George. I'm surprised he's still with us." I take a sip of coffee and look up at Jason.

"What's up with him?"

"A daughter's shown up. She wants the DNR reversed."

I almost sputter coffee on the page. "What?"

"Yes. We've talked to her, but ..." Jason shrugs.

"Didn't know he had a daughter."

"Nobody did. She flew in from the States last night."

"Seriously? She wants the DNR reversed?"

"Yup. Good luck." Jason wanders away, plunks himself in a chair, and starts tapping on a keyboard.

I sigh and sit at the counter. Before I talk to the surprise visitor, I'd better make sure I get all my facts straight. I open the tome, take a gulp of coffee, and start to skim.

George is a seventy-four-year-old man with oesophageal cancer. He's a retired truck mechanic who lives alone after a divorce. He's also a heavy smoker and drinker. A few months ago, he began having episodes of food regurgitation. As time went on, he had increasing trouble swallowing and began to lose weight. A scope showed a tumour in his lower oesophagus. Through the scope, it looked like a hydra, with tentacles fluttering in the central cavity of the oesophagus. A biopsy showed adenocarcinoma, a cancer arising from the glandular tissue.

Adenocarcinoma: from *adeno*, the Greek for gland. Along with squamous cancers, the most common type of cancer in the human body. *Squames* erupt as lumps or sores from the lining cells of ducts and passages, while adenocarcinomas are subterranean creatures arising from deeper pouches and sacs that form and contain bodily secretions.

Scans showed George's cancer to be deeply embedded in adjacent tissues, with at least one root curled round the aorta. As in Betty's and Tom's cases, a surgeon declared the cancer inoperable and sent him on for radiation.

He was admitted to our ward two months ago for nutritional support and to formulate a plan for treatment. He was to receive a combination of external radiation and brachytherapy, the latter involving placing an applicator loaded with radioactive sources in the oesophagus – a modern version of a very old radiation technique involving a "radium bougie" slid into the oesophagus.

Before he could receive any treatment, his condition deteriorated. As so often happens, cancer raced ahead of medical intervention. His swallowing got worse, and a repeat scan showed the hydra had grown. Its tentacles had knotted into a lump which now obstructed the oesophageal passage to a degree far too narrow to place the applicator for radiation. A tube placed in the stomach through the abdominal wall bypassed the blockage, so George's nutrition could be maintained. Worst of all, repeat scans showed the beast had colonized the rest of his body. Dark blotches of metastases appeared in the lungs, liver, and bones.

The previous plan for radiation had given George a slim chance of cure, but now his disease was clearly incurable. The goal of treatment became palliation – relief of symptoms. He received a short course of external radiation which did nothing other than make his remaining swallowing ability painful from radiation oesophagitis. He was seen by a medical oncologist, who ruled out chemotherapy because of his poor condition. It was a classic Catch-22 of oncology: the patient's cancer made him too ill to receive treatment for the cancer causing the illness in the first place. George was given increasingly fancy cocktails of narcotics, steroids, and nerve blockers, all of which only partially relieved his pain.

His uncontrolled pain, together with the lack of anyone to care for him at home, prevented him from leaving hospital, so he stayed on our ward, waiting, waiting ... waiting for what? A miracle? Spontaneous regression? Arrival of a long-lost relative to care for him at home? A bed in the palliative care unit? None of these happened. The palliative care doctor made a quick visit and decided not to admit him to her unit. She felt there was nothing she could do that we weren't doing already.

Over the weeks, I watched helplessly as his once muscular body, consumed by the ravenous monster within, shrank to the classic form of cancer cachexia – sunken, dull eyes, cheeks hollowed to dark pits, muscles wasted so his skin became a gauzy drapery over the skeleton. I also saw his previously cheerful demeanour give way, in the face of relentless pain, futile procedures, and loneliness, to a profound weariness – a weariness common in end-stage cancer patients.

A couple of weeks ago, I'd paid a visit and found him, as I usually did, a shrivelled forlorn figure, lying under blankets in an unfolded recliner. His head, surmounted with a frayed brown toque, poked from the top of the blankets. There was the low thump of reggae from a battered boom box on his night table. He gazed out the window into a barren inner courtyard.

I followed the direction of his gaze and glimpsed Death seated in a corner of the courtyard, quietly puffing on a cigarette.

George's head slowly swivelled towards me, and he looked me directly in the eyes. "Doc, I don't think I can take this anymore," he said.

It was the invitation I needed to discuss his code status.

Like cancer departments, hospitals are run by protocols, scripts. The script for the scenario of the failure of a patient's heart or lungs is Code Blue: a summons for a medical team to swoop in like Valkyries to perform resuscitation. The team attempts to revive the patient using CPR, oxygen, IV drugs, intubation (placement of a breathing tube in the windpipe), and those electric paddles so dear to the hearts of writers of TV dramas. If these initial measures are successful, the patient is transferred to the ICU for further recovery, including assisted breathing – known colloquially as life support.

I've never been sure of the historical origins of this universal policy. It possibly originated from fear of legal reprisal in the situation in which someone with a reversible condition was not revived and died by mistake. Yet its routine application to all patients, especially dying cancer patients, has long been recognized as illogical, if not absurd. Studies show the futility of CPR and ICU care to extend the lives and improve the comfort of terminally ill cancer patients. Quite the opposite: attempts at resuscitation – which produce such nasty effects as broken ribs and a bruised windpipe – often exacerbate suffering. I've seen many cancer patients linger for days in the ICU, their bodies kept alive by pumps and infusions until inevitable death. For patients like George, a quiet delivery into the waiting arms of Death is a welcome alternative.

The persistence of the routine Code Blue is tied to hospitals' self-image as places where only cure and recovery occur, where Death is invisible. As their glossy marketing materials for fundraising campaigns show, hospitals project a heroic, relentlessly upbeat attitude. The "failure" of a patient's heart or lungs – a.k.a. death – is taboo. This attitude helps to explain why the establishment of palliative care units, wards for the care of the terminally ill where dying is acknowledged, has often encountered resistance. In every hospital I've ever worked in, including George's, palliative care beds remain in short supply. Traditionally, hospitals have invested more resources in glamourous technologies directed towards sophisticated treatments than in places some disparagingly call "death wards."

The only way to overwrite the Code Blue script is to replace it with a DNR order. For George, I'd have to initiate a discussion and obtain his consent. Once signed, the DNR flag would be placed on his chart, a warning to all his caregivers that he's not to be resuscitated if one or more of his vital organs fail.

Calling a Code on George would be utterly futile. His plaintive tone told me he was ready for the end.

Yet as I fetched the blank DNR form from the desk, returned to his room, and pinned it to his chart, I was filled with anxiety.

For one thing, I have to bring up the subject of death with him. I'm as culturally conditioned as anyone in finding the topic of death unpalatable. Like the C-word, the D-word is one of those fishbone words that stick in the throat. Yes, George, Death is sitting in the courtyard, waiting for you. Here's your death warrant. Please sign here.

My anxiety is tied to the heroic attitude inculcated in me in medical school and reinforced by the hospital environment. DNR means failure. The Code would have been the last resort, the end of the line, the final possible treatment; if I withdraw it, there's nothing left but abject failure. Signing the patient over to Death feels like a colossal betrayal of my profession, the supposed vanquisher of Death.

Yet here on this ward, crammed with dying patients, the results of medical failure are everywhere. Treatments fail, and patients die all the time. Opening the door to a peaceful death in someone with an incurable disease: Is that really failure? In similar circumstances, surely all of us wish for a quiet, comfortable passing, away from the hubbub and discomfort of the ICU. Isn't part of medical practice knowing when to let go? Against the tide of heroic activism, isn't providing a patient with a gentle departure a success? Shouldn't hospitals be places of comfort as well as cure?

I looked up and met George's gaze. I resorted to a familiar line, honed from previous discussions with terminally ill patients.

"Uh, I don't want to frighten you, but have you thought about what you want done if your heart stops beating or your lungs stop working?"

George raised his head and stared at me.

"You mean die?"

I was momentarily stunned by the ease with which the D-word sprang from his throat.

"Erm ... I guess, yes."

"Oh, for God's sake please don't put me on life support. Just let me go peacefully."

I nod. "If I was in your position, I'd do the same."

I explained what the DNR decision entailed and offered the form for his signature. His hand faltered, and his signature was a wobbly scrawl. But it was enough.

Back at the desk, I wrote a note inside his chart about our exchange, and handed the chart to a nurse. When she saw the DNR flag, she nodded and smiled in silent approval.

Everything seemed to be in place for this man to die without heroic efforts to save him.

Until today. Now, this bright Sunday morning, I enter Room 477. There's the familiar muffled thump of the reggae. One glance at George tells me he's actively dying. He's in bed, propped up on a heap of pillows, his head rotated to one side, mouth a gaping black hole, eyes dark slits. The toque has slipped to one side, covering one ear. An oxygen tank blasts at full power, but his belly still heaves in and out with the effort to draw air into his lungs through a plastic mask.

I tap him gently on the shoulder. "George. George." Despite several taps of increasing firmness, he doesn't react. I draw open his eyelids. His pupils are dull black dots, lifeless, unseeing.

A tall figure rises from a corner seat.

"Good morning."

It's a middle-aged woman wearing a navy power suit with large wing-like lapels. Her hair sweeps up and back in a steely helmet with bronze highlights. She snaps off the boom box.

"I'm his daughter, Sandra."

"Oh. Hi. I'm Dr. Hayter. Uh ... I didn't know he had a daughter."

"Here I am. I flew in last night."

She nods towards her father.

"So what are you going to do, doctor?"

"Can we talk?"

I beckon and lead her outside into the space between two linen carts in the corridor.

"I'm sorry to tell you your dad's dying."

"Anyone can see that. We can't let that happen."

"Erm ... he's got advanced cancer. There's really nothing more we can do other than keep him comfortable."

"What? You can't just let him die. The nurse said you're a radiation doctor. Why aren't you giving him radiation?'

"We did, but nothing happened."

"Then give him more."

"Uh ... I don't think that's a good idea."

Her heels click as she takes a step towards me. The lapels seem to flutter. I lurch back against a pile of blankets.

"Are you saying you're giving up on him?"

"He's in no condition for more radiation."

"My doctors would never give up."

She notices my puzzled look.

"I'm the VP, finance, of a hospital in Maryland. We have a world-class cancer department. Our doctors never give up. If this is what Canadian healthcare is like, I sure hope I don't get sick while I'm up here."

Inwardly, I hope I don't end up on life support in a hospital in Maryland.

I take a big breath.

"I'm sorry. Your father's dying. We'll keep him as comfortable as we can."

"No. I want everything possible done to keep him alive."

"Everything?"

"Radiation, breathing machines, life support, the works."

"Sorry, but those aren't your father's wishes."

"Bullshit. My dad's a fighter."

I pull the chart from under my arm.

"Look. Here's his DNR. We have his signature."

She snatches the form and studies it.

"No way. That's not his."

She hands it back. I have to admit the scrawl is almost indecipherable.

"Well, he was weak the day he signed it. I witnessed it."

"Even if it is his, it's not worth the paper it's written on. He's snowed from all the meds he's on. How could he know what he was signing?"

"He needs those meds to keep his pain under control. The day he signed he was alert and capable of making his own decisions."

She takes another sharp step towards me. Those lapels are about to whap me on the ears.

"Are you listening to me? I want this goddamn Death Order rescinded. I want everything done."

I lean back against the stack of blankets. I feel a strong impulse to bury myself inside.

I study her angry face. If you're so concerned about your father, why didn't you come earlier? Why weren't you involved in the important previous decisions? Why did you wait until this moment of crisis?

"It's not so easy," I say. "Your father has cancer in many parts of his body. Trying to resuscitate someone like this is futile."

"How many times do I need to say it? You - can't - just - give - up," she says, punctuating each word with a jab of a gleaming fingertip.

"It's not giving up. It's just facing reality. Reviving your dad and sending him to the ICU would just prolong his suffering. Do you want that?"

The word suffering disarms her, and she steps back.

I right myself. For a moment we stand face to face, staring into each other's eyes, surrounded by a discordant symphony of beeps, buzzes, intercom broadcasts, cries for help, and moans.

I take a deep breath and try to see things from her viewpoint. She's flown in to find her father on his deathbed. Perhaps she's riddled with guilt over neglecting him these past few weeks. Perhaps there's some unfinished business holding her back from letting him go.

My inner rational doctor knows the patient's wishes, not his daughter's, are paramount and the DNR directive should be respected. But he signed it two weeks ago, and patients' wishes can change. Occasionally, to everyone's surprise a patient's condition improves to the point where they rescind the DNR order. George's condition has deteriorated, but maybe if he saw his estranged daughter, he might perk up and ask for a bit more time. I wish he was well enough to confirm his wishes in front of her. Today, he's far beyond the point of expressing anything at all.

Her face softens.

"Look. Have you any idea what this is like? I haven't seen my father for twelve years. I just want to spend time with him. Please do something. Are you a doctor or a fucking robot?"

A constricted gurgle emanates from George's room.

We rush into the room. Like many cancer patients at this stage, he's momentarily alert. It's as if the brain makes one last attempt to prevent being pulled under into the ocean of oblivion. He's wriggling forward, trying to sit up. His eyes flutter open and he sees his daughter.

"Sandra," he croaks.

She goes to the bedside and grasps his hand.

"Dad. Sit back. Relax."

George slumps back on the pillows. They gaze into each other's eyes.

"It's been so long. How's your mom?" he whispers.

"Good. She sends you her best."

He smiles and she turns to me.

"Please, please. I just can't let him die."

Her words emerge in a desperate childlike whine. The sound drives deep into my soul, striking a chord of sympathy, stirring my memories of the missed opportunities for connection with my father before he died. An urge to help her shoves my resistance aside.

I leave the room and stride to the nursing station. I plunk the chart on the counter, rip the DNR form off, and write "Full Code" in the orders. I shove it towards Jason.

He gasps. "You gotta be kidding," he says.

My cheeks burn. I may have helped Sandra, but I sure haven't helped the nurses, who will bear the brunt of trying to revive a dying man. They'll have to deal with the awful cracking of ribs during CPR, the choking and flying mucous as the breathing tube slides in, the spattered blood from needles. They'll hate me forever for this.

"Sorry."

The other nurses drop their work and gather in a line on the other side of the counter. Their incredulous gazes shift between lunatic me and the Full Code order.

One of them, a young woman in baby blue scrubs, pipes up.

"Okay, doctor, how about a Slow Code?"

Slow Code is a term for a controversial procedure where the nurses go through the motions of a Full Code, but at a slow, gentle pace. They may not even call the full hospital code team. It's a ritual performed for the benefit of the family, considered by many to be unethical because it violates patients' wishes.

"She'll see through that," I say. "She's a bigwig in a hospital in the States."

Bev, a tough older nurse with a face etched from years of dealing with difficult patients and even more difficult doctors, elbows her way through the line.

"Call Charlie Rice."

Dr. Charlie Rice is a senior internal medicine doctor, in charge of the ICU, who's on duty today. He's the gatekeeper to the ICU, where George will end up if he is by some miracle resuscitated. The last person Dr. Rice and his staff want is a dying cancer patient blocking an ICU bed useful for someone with a reversible condition – say, a young victim of an automobile accident. All doctors are gatekeepers to finite resources, and just as I have the right to refuse radiation for a patient, he has a right to say no to the admission of a patient to the ICU if he feels the expensive resources would be futile or wasted. And if Charlie says no to the ICU, then there's clearly no point in calling a Code.

It's a logical plan. But as Bev stares at me, waiting for a response, an ugly feeling nibbles at me: pride. A summons to Dr. Price would be tantamount to an admission I can't handle the situation myself. Doctors are trained to be independent thinkers, capable of making decisions alone. It's an admission of weakness, even ineptitude, to call in a colleague for a situation like this. Other medical specialists, especially internists, already have a dim view of the medical abilities of radiation oncologists, and I don't want to give them more fodder for their opinions.

But I need help. I reign in my hubris and nod. Bev calls Dr. Rice.

A few minutes later, he strides onto the ward, accompanied by a phalanx of junior doctors, bright white coats fluttering around their calves. He's a short, beefy man with the erect bearing of a Marine sergeant. Today, he's wearing a tight pink golf shirt stretched over a bulging breast-plate of pecs.

"What's up?" he barks.

I fill him in on the situation. As I recount George's story, his steely grey eyes bore into me. I can't help reading contempt in his expression. Why is this Rad Onc wasting my time? Doesn't he have the guts to handle this himself? My voice begins to quaver like a second-year medical student being drilled about a case.

Before I finish, he interrupts.

"I'll deal with it," he snaps, and marches directly to George's room, followed by his team.

The nurses and I watch the white-coated phalanx disappear into 477. How is he going to handle Sandra? I decide to follow. Before I can enter, Dr. Price and his team emerge. He thrusts George's chart into my arms.

"There you go," he says, and like a company of soldiers who've just performed a swift deadly strike, he and his team sweep from the ward.

I open the chart. He's scrawled: "Not a candidate for the ICU. **DNR.**"

What happened in that room? How did Dr. Price do what I couldn't do? Did he make Sandra back down? And how did he do it so quickly? His technique must be efficient, almost brutal, likely honed through years of speaking to families in the fraught environment of the ICU. For a moment I'm envious of his skill and his guts. But did he also recognize Sandra's pain and longing?

I carry the chart back to the desk and lay it open at the page showing the new DNR order. Bev glances at it. She gives me a slightly haughty, triumphant smile.

"Thanks for your help, Bev," I say.

The nurses scatter and resume their work. I'm getting behind seeing the other patients. As I pull another chart from the rack, I think: I hope Sandra is getting the time she wants with her father.

A chime rings. The nurses and I glance at the display. It's 477.

"Uh-oh," Jason mutters.

Jason and I trot to 477.

George's lifeless body slumps over one side of the bed. Sandra's quivering form hunches in a bedside chair. She's still gripping her father's hand.

The room is still, quiet, dark. Death's pall has descended. I hear only the incessant hiss of the open oxygen line and Sandra's muffled sobs.

15

The Desperate Couple

By the time I arrive in Calgary, it's too late.

My father has fallen into the clutches of a urologist - not the senior Brit who gave him his hormone treatment, but a young hotshot who, without explaining other options, has stabbed his back and thrust rubber tubes directly into the kidneys to bypass the blockage by the cancer. My father's kidney function has improved, and he's become more alert.

Damn. I hate this reflex behaviour of performing a technical procedure in a dying cancer patient without considering the bigger context. The drainage tubes are only a stopgap measure. They will buy my father time, but sooner or later some new crisis will occur - then another, and another. Crisis will follow crisis on a stuttering downward slope. Death patiently waits at the bottom with open arms. Time spent on this rickety one-way roller coaster is rarely good quality time.

Medical students and residents - mesmerized as they are by technological wizardry - are always keen to do procedures, but I always caution them that just because a procedure *can* be done, that does not mean it *should* be done. In a dying patient without hope of cure, the option of masterful inactivity should always be put on the menu.

So quick and reactive were the urologist's actions, my father was given no chance to review the menu. In any case, it turns out he and my mother have never discussed his wishes around medical intervention. Like me, they have long known this moment was coming but have chosen to ignore it, like it's some distant mirage. The scrim of silence descended again.

By the time I arrive at my father's bedside in a small, dark room in a remote corner of Calgary General Hospital, the drainage tubes are a fait accompli. I see no point in stirring things up. It's far easier to prevent an intervention than reverse it.

He lies under blankets on the bed, sleeping, an IV dripping in one arm, an oxygen mask flopping at his jaw, murky amber liquid coursing through tubes from his flanks to drainage bags slung under the bed.

My mother sits at his bedside in a wheelchair – all the stress has made her lupus act up. She rolls forward and pats my father's arm.

"Look who's here to see you."

He rouses, raises his head from the pillow, and looks at me. Through the rectangular frames of his glasses, his eyes are clouded, dull. His lips curve in a weak smile.

"Oh. Hello," he says, in a chirpy matter-of-fact tone, like I've been gone only a few hours on some errand.

For the first time since his diagnosis, he looks truly sick. Cachexia, wasting, is underway. His cheeks have sunk to dark pits, and his once-thick black hair is thin and streaked with silver. Purple-grey blotches mottle his arms. A film of sweat glistens on his broad forehead.

These features are those of a hundred dying cancer patients I've attended to. This time, it's my father.

He spots something on the wall behind me.

"There's that woman again."

I turn to a faded framed print depicting a forest with a row of bright red poppies in the foreground. A typical example of hospital art that's meant to cheer you up, but instead provokes queasiness.

"I don't see any woman."

"She's there. Hiding behind that tree. She's looking at me! Go away! Go away!" he shouts.

The renal toxins are still affecting his brain. I take the picture from the wall, flip it, and place it on the floor. My father's head falls back, and within a few minutes he's asleep again.

My mother and I spend the next couple of days at my father's bedside. We watch him sleep. We wait, wait, and wait some more for something to happen. For me at work, hospitals are busy, frenetic places, where I constantly scurry here and there to perform a never-ending list of tasks. Now, from a patient's point of view, everything seems to unfold in the slowest of slow motion. I understand the frustrations of families waiting to see me.

Visits by a nurse to take his vital signs or check his tubes punctuate the long periods of inactivity and waiting. Occasionally, his urologist – a curly-haired, boyish-faced man who turns out to be a former medical school classmate of mine – pops his head around the edge of the door like Mr. Punch peering around the wings of a puppet show. "Everything okay?" he asks peremptorily, then immediately disappears. His manner recalls the evasive behaviour of surgeons I'd first witnessed with Sam.

Brandishing her stick with the retractable claw, my mother reminds everyone who comes into the room that my father's a Senior Doctor, she's a former Nurse, and always introduces me as "my Son, the Doctor, a Specialist." But these hijinks don't elicit any special treatment, just polite smiles.

My mother and I spend the evenings at the house. As we sit side by side on the sofa, soothing the numbness from the inertia of the hospital with the flickering TV screen, my mother, without prompting, begins to talk about the disappointments in her marriage. I suppose the threat of her husband's death has provoked reflection on their life together. Early in their marriage, she wanted him to abandon his thoughts of becoming a specialist and instead become a GP. They would settle down in a quiet village nestled in the English countryside where he could operate his practice from a "surgery" adjacent to a large family home spilling over with children and pets, all presided over by her. My father's determination to become a specialist, which resulted in long hours of work and study away from home, and abortive attempts to gain a foothold on the cruel career ladder of British specialty medicine, shattered this idyllic dream. While he was in training, they had trouble making ends meet, and she had to take part-time jobs as a night nurse in a nursing home and in a jam factory. She mimes the act of plucking the leaves off strawberries with angry vehemence, then abruptly shifts to comic mode as she crams invisible fruit into her mouth like Lucy gobbling chocolates on the candy line. After my father finished his training, his rejection from a post in London was the springboard to move to Canada, a move that wrenched my mother from her beloved home country and extended family. In Winnipeg, she was so homesick for England she wanted to move back almost immediately. As she relates her story, I hear a resentful undertone common to all women forced to give up their own dreams in favour of their husbands' careers.

On the third morning I decide to chase Mr. Punch into the corridor outside my father's room.

"Hey, Jake. So how do you think my dad is doing?"

"Temp's normal," he says with a bright smile. "His creatinine's come way down." Creatinine is a marker of kidney function.

Yeah, I think, his creatinine's better, but the cancer is worse. I recognize a common phenomenon, of which I've sometimes been guilty: focusing on improvements in technicalities, such as lab data, to provide a false sense of optimism in a dire situation.

Obviously proud it's his plumbing work that's led to the improvement, he gives me a satisfied smirk and turns away.

"Uhh ... Can I ask what the plan is?" The word "plan" catches him short. He stops and turns.

"Plan?"

I take a big breath. "It's pretty clear his cancer's getting worse."

"Oh, yeah, that," he says, like I've reminded him of some trivial detail. "We'll get the med onc to see him about some chemotherapy." He scurries away.

At the time of my father's illness, chemotherapy for advanced prostate cancer is next to useless, an opinion confirmed by the medical oncologist, a middle-aged woman with an aristocratic demeanour, adorned with a stylish dress and pearls like she's ready for a night at the opera.

As I expected, she punts the situation forward.

"He's in no shape to get chemo now, my dear," she says, laying a bejewelled, manicured hand on my arm.

"I'll book him to see me again in a month. We can revisit the situation then. Have a wonderful day."

There's a slim chance my father will be alive in a month. It's that Catch-22 again. Too sick to get treatment that might help the disease causing the sickness. Her delay is just a tactic to disengage without appearing to disengage. She releases my arm, gives me a sort of curtsey, and slides away.

I watch her receding figure disappear. As I stand alone in the corridor, brushed by passing nurses, surrounded by the familiar hospital cacophony of beeps, blips, buzzes, moans, and shouts, anger at her abrupt, uninterested manner – and that of my father's urologist – rises inside me. Why the hell don't they care? Why are they running away? Why are they writing him off? Why aren't they doing more to help my father? To save him?

My logical, scientific doctor's approach to my father's situation suddenly crumbles against a tide of desperation. How can my father be allowed to die? At sixty-six, he's young enough to look forward to a few more decades of active life. To enjoy his retirement. To travel back to his birthplace, India. To see parts of the world he hasn't visited. To see his grandchildren grow up.

I want to shout help. *Help.* Why isn't anyone doing anything? Can someone please do something?

Surely, there must be something, somewhere, to rescue him, bring him back, give him more time – time for me to achieve that reconciliation I crave.

~

One glance at Cindy told me she was dying.

Propped up on pillows, she lay on an unfolded sofa bed in the living room of the townhouse she shared with her husband, Jim. Clusters of enlarged lymph nodes poked out from under her jaw. I couldn't help thinking of a greedy chipmunk, jowls stuffed with food – but Cindy's swellings were feeding on her, reducing her to yet another of those pale cadaveric figures familiar from the hospital wards.

It was almost impossible to reconcile this sick, frail person with the memory of a vibrant, powerful woman, once short-listed for Canada's Olympic gymnastics team. Most recently, she'd been my daughter's gymnastics coach and a family friend. "Go, go, go!" she'd yell from the sidelines, as she pushed her team to greater, higher feats.

Here she was, at age thirty-six, on the final lap of a two-year run with lymphoma, a cancer of the lymphatic system. Her disease had progressed relentlessly despite repeated assaults with chemotherapy and radiation. A month ago, her lymphoma specialist uttered the fateful words "I have nothing more to offer you."

As I approached, she looked up at me and smiled. Ivory bone shone through the translucent membrane of skin covering her forehead. Her emaciation gave a new, childlike prominence to her soft blue eyes.

"It's good to see you," she croaked. The lymph nodes must be pressing on her larynx.

She extended her hand, and I grasped it lightly. Her fingers were as cold as metal pipes.

"So, how are you doing?" I heard my voice lapse into the falsely cheerful tone I'd often used at the bedside of my own patients.

"Great!" she replied, echoing my upbeat tone with a coach's enthusiasm.

"She sure is." I heard a gruff voice behind me. I turned to see Jim, a stocky man in his midthirties with the square build of a linebacker.

He came forward and smiled at his wife. "She's not going to let this lick her – are you, hon?"

"No way!"

Jim looked pale, and around his dark-brown eyes, I saw tiny creases that betrayed the fatigue of caring for Cindy.

"Thanks for coming over," he said. "We need your help."

"Sure," I said.

Jim went to the kitchen and returned with a small glass vial. He thrust it at me.

"Can you give this to her?"

"What is it?" I asked.

"714X. Amazing treatment for lymphoma. We found it on the Internet."

I frowned. "Huh. Never heard of it."

"Figured. You doctors don't know half of what's out there."

"Can I take a look?"

I took the vial and held it up to the light. An oily liquid shimmered behind the amber glass. I rotated the vial and the liquid emitted gold sparkles. I noticed Cindy gazing at it like it was holy water.

"Any idea what's in it?"

"Nope. But we checked on the Internet, and boy, does it ever work. Can you give it to her? It needs to be injected right into one of her swollen nodes."

"Uh ... I'm not sure."

"Come on. Didn't they teach you to give needles in medical school?"

"Yes, but ..."

"Everything's ready." He pointed to a syringe on a side table.

"I'm sorry, but ..."

"But what?" Jim drew back his shoulders and stepped towards me.

"I've no idea what's in it or if it works."

"Come on. We thought you were our friend."

There was silence as Jim and Cindy stared at me. My gaze fell to the tangle of sheets at the end of the bed.

After a moment I said, "Tell you what. Let me do a bit of homework on this stuff."

Jim shrugged. "Fair enough. Don't be too long about it. She's going downhill fast."

When I stepped through Cindy and Jim's front door that evening, I crossed a physical and a professional boundary. Doctors are not supposed to offer medical advice or treatment to anyone other than their own patients. This unwritten code exists partly because it could be misleading or even downright dangerous to offer advice to someone without having examined them or reviewed their test results. An opinion constructed on the basis of a casual conversation might change if I had access to the facts. In addition, I don't want to say anything to undermine the care the person is already receiving from their regular doctor.

Yet, as any doctor will attest, requests for medical advice from friends and family members are very common. It's yet another occupational hazard they don't teach you about in medical school. As an oncologist, I'm a prime target for such requests. It's not uncommon for someone at a social gathering to sidle up to me and say, "My aunt has [insert type of] cancer. They're recommending [insert name of random treatment]. What do you think?" or, worse still, ask me to *look* at something on their body. I arrived home one evening to find Sal, our hypochondriac neighbour, barring the way to the front door, mouth open, pointing to a wart on her tongue. At a gay men's retreat, I was lured into a side room by an elderly church organist who wanted me to examine a "pimple" on his scrotum. On one level, these requests are just plain annoying. Most people must know oncology is a demanding field and the last thing I want to talk about at a party or on vacation.

All through my career I've struggled to deflect such requests with various degrees of success. I can brush off strangers like the person at a party with a smile and "I really can't comment without knowing all the details" or "I'm sure she's in good hands," or the church organist with "You should get your own doctor to look at that."

Sometimes the best approach is to stay closeted. A psychiatrist friend once told me he tells people he's a landscape gardener – not a complete lie, as he is a very talented gardener, not just a whacker of mental weeds. I sometimes tell people at social gatherings I'm a writer. But it becomes hard to stay quiet when I'm witness to conversations about medical care, especially when the conversations contain inaccuracies about treatments. Then, I can't avoid the urge to set the record straight. In my play *Lady-in-Waiting*, the main character is a doctor with a secret life as a drag queen. When one of her drag colleagues falls seriously ill, the boundary between Kandi's worlds crumbles. The separation of professional and personal identities is a struggle for all professions, but the stakes are particularly high in medicine.

Subterfuge or deflection are much harder with close friends or immediate family members. I care about these people, and they're in my life for the long term. I sense their confusion and fear. I understand how helpful it can be to know someone who can help interpret the cancer jargon and paint the big picture. With these folks, I often use broad brushstrokes rather than discuss the details of a personal situation. I'm also happy to clarify terminology, especially when it comes to radiation, and very happy when I'm able to bust my pet-peeve myth about "burning."

On a few occasions, I've arranged second opinions for friends with specialists I trust. These requests sometimes give me a window into the brusque manner with which colleagues can treat patients. A friend may say something like "I just don't like Dr. X. He's a cold fish and never spends any time with me. Can you find me someone else?" I don't like to undermine colleagues, but I recognize the added tension of staying in a relationship with a disliked doctor. I always encourage friends to be open about changes with the original doctor.

As in Cindy and Jim's case, the requests from friends often take the form of questions about alternative or unconventional therapies. "Hey, doc, what do you think about shark cartilage for my cancer?"

Cindy and Jim's situation presented a brand-new twist on this familiar scenario. They weren't just asking for advice: they were asking me to administer a treatment.

As soon as I got home that evening, I sat at the computer and googled "714X." It turned out to have been around for a very long time, since the 1960s, when a Quebec doctor came up with the idea of preventing cancer cells from trapping nitrogen needed for their growth by administering camphor, a substance derived from an evergreen tree found in Asia. Yes, I remembered the massive, shady *kampur* trees in the Singapore Botanic Gardens and the plaque about the use of its resin in medicine. In fact, camphor has a long history of medicinal use in countries such as India and China. It the West, it was once an ingredient in paregoric, an opium-camphor mixture for diarrhoea. Today it is still found in a topical chest rub for cold symptoms.

But camphor was one of those remedies that never successfully moved from the fringes to the mainstage of medicine. There was no scientific proof it had any effect on cancer. Like Peter's Prostacure, there were lots of testimonials from cancer patients – "The cure I was looking for!" "The miracle treatment doctors don't want you to know about!" – but none of these claims were backed up by robust clinical trials. The US FDA disapproved of the use of 714X for any condition, and in fact banned its import into the United States.

But as with other alternative medicines, a black market persisted. I located the website of a company distributing 714X through online sales. I guessed this was where Cindy and Jim obtained their supply. Two small vials cost close to $500.00. Cindy and Jim were not well off, and their $500.00 could have been better spent elsewhere. I felt a surge of anger at the faceless entrepreneur who was getting rich off vulnerable cancer patients like her.

From this quick review, I could see 714X was yet another in a long line of bogus treatments for cancer marketed to desperate cancer patients. No way could I participate in such quackery.

Just to be sure, I called my colleague Dr. Tsang, who could always be counted on for a sound, reasonable opinion. As soon as I mentioned 714X, his tone turned dismissive.

"714X? Yeah, I've heard of it. Total bullshit. You know the crackpot who came up with it lost his medical licence?"

That night I lay in bed, staring into the darkness. I liked Cindy and Jim, and wanted to help them. I didn't want Cindy to die. She was a lovely person, generous, open, warm-hearted with lots to offer the world. She'd helped my daughter's fitness and self-confidence. I didn't want to lose her.

Like Peter, Cindy was an adult, free to do what she liked with her body. I believed in the right of competent patients to choose what's done to them. If I gave the injection, I'd just be helping her do what she wanted.

And who knows? Maybe 714X works. Were all those testimonials groundless? Medical history shows many substances, radium included, were accepted as efficacious only after a period of profound scepticism. Serendipitous discoveries often make their way to the mainstage of medicine. In my lifetime, the cause of stomach ulcers changed from "stress" to infection through the surprise discovery of bacteria in the stomach. Perhaps someone needed to conduct a proper clinical trial of 714X. Hah – maybe I could start a trial, with Cindy as the first patient.

At that thought, my inner doctor woke up and wagged his finger at me. Look, isn't Cindy's desire for 714X just denial? If you give the injection, you'll be colluding in delusion when they should be facing reality. Cindy should be settling her affairs and preparing for death.

And, doctor, do you really know what's in that vial? What if it's laced with toxins? What if something goes wrong? What if she has bad side effects? You could be charged with malpractice and have your licence revoked. Dr. Tsang's reminder that the inventor of 714X lost his licence echoed.

I felt anger again at the unscrupulous, uncaring businessman who'd already made money off Cindy and Jim.

No. I had to refuse. My mind made up, I settled into my pillow.

After I pulled my car up outside Jim and Cindy's house the following evening, I turned off the engine and sat for a few minutes. I gazed into the silent, dark street and tried to contain the anxiety around breaking my decision.

A sleek black wagon was parked on the other side of the street. From above the steering wheel, Death grinned at me.

Inside, Cindy, looking even more like a limp doll, was propped up on the pillows. Jim stood at her side like a sentry. As I entered, they stared at me expectantly.

"Well?" said Jim.

I looked him square in the eyes.

"Sorry. I can't do it. I can't find any evidence it works."

"Come on. Tons of people say they've been cured."

"Just anecdotes – not backed up by any science. There's even no proof any of them had cancer. If you really want this, maybe you can find someone else."

"The GP's washed his hands. We asked Cindy's sister, a nurse, but she's scared of complications."

"Well, I am too."

"How can there be complications? It's totally natural."

"Sometimes these so-called natural products have harmful ingredients. And needles can cause bleeding, infection."

"I don't care. I just want to live," Cindy croaked.

I sat on the edge of the sofa bed and took her hand. I looked into her big, luminous eyes and saw again the beautiful, strong, kind person she had once been. I wanted so much to help her. I had to forget she was a friend. Lines I'd used with my patients ticker-taped across my mind.

"I know this is hard, but I don't think there's any treatment against the cancer that will do you good. The important thing now is to focus on your comfort and plan how you want to spend the rest of your days. I can arrange a palliative care doctor who can –"

Jim grabbed my shoulder.

"Stop. She's not ready for that."

I gently removed his hand from my shoulder and stood up.

"If there's anything you need, please let me know."

"We told you what we need," grunted Jim.

I headed for the door.

"*Please!*"

Cindy's voice stopped me. Her hoarse, desperate cry struck a primal chord deep inside me, the instinct to survive shared by all human beings. *Help me. I don't want to die.* It nudged awake another instinct: the doctor's reflex to do something, anything, to preserve life.

Some kind of invisible, irresistible force took over. I plucked the vial from the table and snapped off its top. The sharp piney scent of camphor wafted into the room. I quickly drew the golden syrup into the syringe.

I asked Cindy to draw up the side of her nightgown. An irregular cluster of lymph nodes protruded from her groin. I plunged the needle through the skin and expelled the liquid into the nodes, and she groaned.

"Sorry," I said.

I asked Jim to put pressure on the area, tossed the syringe aside, strode to the door, then turned with the stiff posture of a Victorian schoolmaster.

"Please don't ask me to do it again. And I'd appreciate it if you could keep this quiet."

"Thank you," Jim called after me.

As I started my car, Death leered at me. I jammed my foot on the accelerator and careened away.

What have you done? You're a Doctor of Medicine, for God's sake. You're supposed to base everything you do on science. What if your colleagues find out? I imagined Dr. Tsang's sneer. "You did what??"

And what if something goes wrong? An allergic reaction, bleeding, infection? Will I get hauled up for malpractice?

I called Jim the next day.

"She's doing great! Thanks again."

I was relieved to hear there'd been no complications. But doing great?

Every time I called over the next few days, I received the same glowing report from Jim.

"You should come see how good she is!"

I found them at the dining room table seated around a giant wheel of pizza in a cardboard carton. It was the first time I'd seen Cindy up and out of the sofa bed. A pizza slice drooped from her bony fingers. She took tentative nibbles from its edges.

"Hey," she said with a bright smile. "Stop gaping and come and sit down. Want some pizza?"

"Thanks, I just ate," I said as I drew up a chair.

Jim munched on pizza. We chatted about the sudden drop in outside temperature heralding winter. As we spoke, I saw a new lustre in Cindy's eyes and heard a new strength in her voice, an echo of her coach's energy. Yet as I looked closer, I also saw signs the disease was advancing: a new clump of nodes peeked from the hollow just above her breastbone.

"Look at how well she's eating," said Jim. "The injection's kicked in."

"Well, I'm glad you're feeling better," I said.

Cindy put down her slice and wobbled to the sofa bed. She lay down and drew up the side of her nightgown.

"How about another shot?"

"Err, I ..."

"She's had no side effects," barked Jim.

I stared at Cindy. My fingers tapped an invisible keyboard on the table. What's going on? She's feeling better. Something's happening. But what? Hamlet's words to Horatio flashed in my mind. *There are more things in heaven and earth than are dreamt of in your philosophy.*

I stood up, strode to her side, and gave the second injection.

A week later, one more. The following week, another.

Each time, she reported improvement in how she felt, but I could see her lymphoma was growing.

On the morning of the day I was scheduled to make the next visit, I was in the middle of a busy clinic when I received an urgent summons to the emergency department.

I drew back the curtain of a tiny cubicle and found Jim, face corrugated in grief, gripping Cindy's lifeless hand. The debris field of a failed resuscitation attempt – tubes, vials, syringes, flecks of blood, and sputum – covered the floor. That morning, he hadn't been able to wake her up. By the time the ambulance arrived at the hospital, it was too late.

I gazed at Cindy's face, now calm, serene as a marble effigy.

My abdominal muscles heaved in a paroxysm of sorrow. "I'm so sorry," I said.

Jim released her hand. He rounded the end of the stretcher, grabbed both my wrists, and stared deeply into my eyes.

"I want to say thank you. You'll never know how much you giving her those injections meant to her. To us. You know, all along we knew 714X was bullshit. Cindy was never a quitter. All she wanted was something to give her hope."

16

The Dying Father

My moment of desperation in the hospital corridor passes. I never seriously consider seeking an unproven remedy for my father. My parents never raise the idea. After all, they're children of twentieth-century scientific medicine and regard anything else as quackery. They view even commonly used procedures such as chiropractic manipulation – which competes with my father's field in treatment of bone and joint disorders – with suspicion and mockery. In addition, the use of Essiac or Laetrile might expose them to the scorn of their many medical friends.

In the absence of any meaningful further treatment for his cancer, the only path forward is acceptance of my father's death. Of course, he's been dying slowly ever since the cancer was diagnosed; the hormone therapy was only a flame retardant. Now, death is imminent. But as the days pass, and my mother and I sit, watch, and wait, we never talk about it. The thick, worn, and frayed curtain of silence descends again. It's a replay of those earlier uncomfortable moments in their garden and on Christmas Eve.

Death is the third member of that Triad of Uncomfortable Subjects – the first two being Cancer Diagnosis and Relapse – poorly prepared for in medical school. The closest I came to formal training was when I worked alongside the social service nurses during my summer placement in oncology. Much of their time was spent trying to help patients and their families accept an impending death. Harder still were their efforts to convince attending doctors to acknowledge the declines of their patients and abandon futile last-ditch treatments. Their pleading didn't always work: I saw moribund patients wheeled under radiation machines in valiant but misguided attempts at heroics.

After I began my practice as an oncologist, where impending death surrounded me, I soon came to recognize the importance of discussing death openly. First, it allows patients to "put their affairs in order," to tidy up the loose ends of their financial and personal affairs, such as getting around to revising that neglected will. Second, as with George, it opens the door to discussions about the intensity of care at the end of life, including the fraught topic of resuscitation. Very often, in the absence of advance directives, children's conflicting views about their parents' care turn into ugly spats at the bedside of a dying parent. If the parent has made his or her wishes known in advance, the family can redirect energy from conflict to a common goal: the parent's comfort. Finally, an acknowledgment of death provides an opportunity for family members and friends to say their farewells – and perhaps to repair broken relationships and gain forgiveness. The ideal is the tableau of the Grand Death, sometimes depicted in art or films, where a parent lies in a big comfy bed, propped up on pillows, surrounded by a crowd of adoring family members, who gaze lovingly as he or she slips away in comfort.

The Grand Death is an elusive ideal. Its attainment is prevented mainly by doctors' and families' resistance to acknowledge and discuss death openly. Many families cling to the idea that discussing death will make the patient "give up" and therefore succumb more quickly. It will also destroy that elusive entity, "hope." In some cultures, the mere utterance of death is considered an ill omen. My partner is of Chinese ancestry, and more than once I've received a sharp jab in the ribs following my faux pas of mentioning death openly in the presence of his family.

But failure to acknowledge the imminence of death leads only to the uncertainty, confusion, and chaos that marked deaths like Cindy's in the emergency room. False hopes of last-ditch cure or miraculous recovery can be replaced by the realistic hope of a peaceful, pain-free death.

In my practice, I'd often relied on the scripts in Buckman's book on breaking bad news to introduce the topic of death. I was sometimes proud of the way I helped families navigate this bewildering and painful subject.

At my father's bedside, I'm inexplicably tongue tied around a subject about which I've done so much reading and reflection. I know I should raise the subject of his death – but I can't do it. I'm stumbling in the footlights like an actor who's "dried" – forgotten his lines in mid-scene.

What's going on? Is it my family's British reserve? Is it that old friend, the imposter syndrome? What gives me the right to talk about his death? Will it make my already high-strung mother even more anxious? Will it rouse the lupus? Will it force my father deeper into his shell? Will it make him angry at me?

Or – is it a personal defence? Am I protecting myself? Would bringing his death into the open force me to acknowledge its reality – and in its wake, the pain of our broken relationship?

As often happens in the third act of a play, a deus ex machina rescues me. As the mental fog of the renal failure lifts, my father's pain returns. In an effort to get comfortable, he constantly twists and turns like he's squirming to avoid some ferocious animal that's crept into bed with him.

I suggest to Jake he call in a palliative care doctor, a specialist in symptom relief, so my father's pain can be better controlled. A palliative care expert can also help my parents make decisions about his future care. Jake gives me a sour look like I've asked him to call an undertaker. He shares the prejudice against palliative care doctors of many of my colleagues, who regard them as the winged harbingers of death and therefore reminders of failure. Patients are easily infected with these attitudes and resist palliative care consultations. But after I point out my father's writhing, Jake agrees. He's glad to shift the responsibility to someone else.

The next morning, as I wheel my mother to the door of my father's room, a short, dapper man in his midfifties, with a bright pink tie and matching silk square poking from his breast pocket, emerges. It's the palliative care doctor.

"Ah! Good morning. I've just been chatting with your dad about *end-of-life care*," he says, with a gleaming smile, like he's been talking to him about buying a shiny new car.

Even palliative care, arguably the most human of all medical fields, has jargon. "End-of-life care" means looking after someone in the process of dying.

"I've asked him to decide whether he wants to die at home or in hospital."

My mother gasps. He's uttered the dreaded, unmentionable D-word, as charged as the C-word.

I barely contain my own gasp. This man's just broken one of the cardinal rules of breaking bad news: Never do it while the patient is alone. Always have a family member present to provide support. Why the hell didn't this slick salesman wait until we arrived? I guess he thinks my dad, a fellow doctor, can take it.

"I've left that with him," he says, like he's left a contract to review. "Can you talk to him about it?"

He smooths his hair and trots away down the hall.

I hesitate at the door. How has my father reacted to this man's bluntness?

I push my mother into the room.

My father hunches on the side of the bed. His body quakes with convulsive sobs. As we enter, he looks up. His face is a mask of agony. Seeing us, he screws his knuckles into his eye sockets, fiercely trying to staunch the flow of tears.

I've never seen my father so small, so frightened. He's a scared, lonely, homesick schoolboy on a bed in the dormitory of that long-ago boarding school.

My mother gestures for me to wheel her forward. She places her hand on his arm.

"Lie down, dear," she says softly.

He gazes at her and sucks in a big gulp of air.

"Why me? Why me? It makes everything so pointless," he whimpers.

He collapses back on the pillow. His torso convulses in more sobs. Tears flood his cheeks.

The spring has finally unwound. All the disappointments and unspoken shames of his life suddenly release, freeing their trapped debris in a maelstrom of raw emotion.

My mother caresses his chest.

"Darling," she says.

I stand flat against the wall, paralysed, helpless. Not even the doctor in me knows how to react or what to say.

The sobs slowly subside. I creep forward, sit on one corner of his bed, and place one hand on his knee. He glances at me, and I smile back. Embarrassed, he folds an arm over his eyes.

Over the next few days, Dr. Pink Pocket Square adjusts my father's painkillers until he is comfortable. He coaxes my parents' wishes for the future from them. My father wants to go home. The doctor arranges for him to be discharged under the care of a community palliative care team who will make home visits.

With his kidney function improved, his pain under better control, and a plan for his care in place, my father's roller coaster car glides to a halt on a plateau. Who knows how long this pause will last? When will the next giddying, frightening drop occur? Maybe days, maybe weeks.

I decide to use the break to go home to catch up on work and spend time with my family.

The evening before I depart, I drive to the hospital to pay a visit to my father on my own.

I sit at his bedside, gazing at his sleeping face. The new, stronger painkillers have made him very drowsy. The only sounds in the room are the hiss of the oxygen apparatus and his soft snores. Outside, the frenzied activity of the daytime has subsided to silence punctuated occasionally by a patient's cry and the bleep of an alarm.

It's just me, my father, and ... where's Death? I half expect to see his dark figure crouching in a corner of the room, or looking over my shoulder at my father with a triumphant grin. He's not anywhere to be seen. In fact, I haven't seen him for a while.

Of course. He's right in front of me. Death is now in my father. Within the frame of my father's body, I can just make out his outline. His white frontal bone glistens beneath the skin of my father's forehead.

This is likely the last time I will see this man who is both father and stranger. The old yearning for connection bubbles up, bringing in its wake a flotsam of regret.

I'm deeply ashamed about the episode in the rec room. A happy family reunion ended in bitter conflict. I called my dying father a bastard. I feel a need to apologize, but shame pushes back. And – am I truly sorry? My father hurt my son. Will an apology be me just acting out once again the respectful, dutiful son?

I can't let my father go to his grave with the word "bastard" ringing in his ears.

Finally, I lean forward and touch my father's arm.

"I just want to say I feel bad about that row we had last year. I'm sorry about the things I said."

My father's eyes blink open. He stares at me for a minute. His mouth opens but no words come out. He lays his right hand on the left side of his chest, then lifts it and points it at me.

I lean over and attempt a hug. My arms wrap his shoulders, and I gently squeeze. He's never been a hugger; greetings and partings were always signalled through a firm handshake. He must recognize this is our final parting. Does he not, as I do, crave some final display of affection? But there's no response.

I squeeze harder and lift him slightly off the bed. Again, no reaction. It's as though he's one of my childhood marionettes, lifted from its box, strings loose, limbs flapping on metal hinges.

Maybe my squeeze has caused pain. Beneath his flesh, his bones are brittle lattice works of cancer. I lay him back, give him one last pat and smile, and leave.

The following morning, which coincides with my fortieth birthday, I fly back east. My wife and kids greet me with a homemade cake and a chorus of "Happy Birthday." My outer cheeriness conceals a deep sadness.

Early evening a month later, at my desk in my office at the cancer centre, I shuffle through a pile of pink slips with telephone messages and try to decide which need to be answered this evening, which tomorrow. The pager strapped to my belt vibrates. That's odd. I'm not on call.

I dial the displayed number, and a man with a Scottish brogue answers. It's Dr. Remington, an acquaintance and former colleague of my father who lives in the same city as me.

"Charles. I just had a call from your mother. I'm sorry to tell you, your father has passed away."

Why has my mother chosen this indirect route for the news? Even in a family crisis, her love of protocol takes over. News of such import should only be conveyed through official channels, doctor to doctor. Very likely too, she wants to avoid calling the house and speaking to the farm girl.

"Thank you for letting me know."

I replace the receiver and stare at the Saliger print. Death leers at me. You've won. That's it. It's over. My father's dead.

I try to summon the tears of a model son, but they just don't come. Right now, there's too much shame, regret, disappointment, and fatigue in the way.

The next morning, the 6:00 a.m. flight to Calgary again. This time, the funeral suit will be used.

At the door of the bungalow, my mother looks pale and puffy, like she's just stepped off a gruelling sixteen-hour flight.

It's late spring, warm enough to sit and have coffee on the patio. Trixie weaves between patches of melting snow, sniffing lustily at the newly bare patches of soil. In one corner, a clump of prairie grass, woken by the spring sun, squeezes its way through a crack in the fence to reclaim its colonized territory.

Without prompting, my mother relates the story of the end.

"Near the end it was very hard. I wanted him to go into the palliative care unit at the hospital, but he refused. I kept telling him it would be best for both of us, but he wouldn't go. So it was up to me to look after him. Because they knew I was a nurse they thought I was up to it. They sent a visiting nurse three times a week, but it was still very hard, looking after him day and night, day and night.

"He was in constant pain. Even the slightest move caused agony, sheer *agony*. The only way for me to deal with it was to give him morphine. I'd mix up a big glass of orange Tang and put a dollop of morphine in it. Towards the end I didn't even measure it or keep track of the doses; I just kept putting dollops in the Tang. No amount was enough. The pain just ran ahead of us.

"The last day I'd given him a glass of Tang, which put him off to sleep. I lay down on the other side of the bed for a nap. All of a sudden, I was woken by this great crash and I saw he'd fallen out of bed. There he was, lying on the floor, stiff as a log, dead. He'd died and just rolled out of bed.

"Of course, I called 911, and the police and fire and ambulance came. The medics worked on him but they couldn't bring him back. The worst thing was, the police said it was an unexpected death so they put up all this yellow tape round the bedroom and I couldn't go in. Imagine that: not being able to see my own dead husband. They called the coroner, who said there'd have to be an autopsy. An autopsy? The man had cancer. Anyway, they bundled him up and carted him off to the morgue."

So much for the Grand Death.

My mother stares at me. She grimaces like a guilty schoolgirl found out with some prank.

"Do you think they think I killed him?"

"Of course not. He was dying of cancer."

My sister arrives from Winnipeg, and my brother, who works in the airline industry, rides in from England on a jump seat in the cockpit of a 767. Both of them look shell-shocked.

At the funeral reception, my father's former colleagues, staff, and patients step up to me one by one to offer condolences. As they grip my hands with earnest looks, they nearly all remark on what a wonderfully warm "people person" my father was. At a funeral nobody is expected to say otherwise, but I'm still taken aback by the sincerity of their affection. My actor's training kicks in: I nod and smile, successfully concealing my surprise at the discrepancy between his professional persona and the remote, shadowy figure I knew at home. The encounters summon a memory of a time I accompanied my father to work when I was a boy and was perplexed by a charm and warmth I rarely saw at home.

It's a dichotomy that feels familiar. Doctoring is the perfect career for getting attention and adulation outside the messy emotional strings of domestic life. Going to work can be a tonic when real intimacy becomes hard. Patients, vulnerable and powerless as they are, often express admiration and gratitude. Oncology, where patients are most vulnerable of all, is fertile ground for this dynamic. My father's field of physical medicine and rehabilitation – dealing with people after devastating events such as amputations and strokes – must be a close runner-up. It's easy to linger at work, go and see one last patient, make one more set of rounds, one more phone call, hear one more "Thank you, doc" to get that fix. It's both addictive and treacherous – treacherous because it's false, based on a persona that operates within a script of professional protocols. The risk lies in allowing this false adulation to replace the challenges of domestic intimacy. I arrive home on a sort of high from the day's encounters, only to have that high rapidly shattered by the need to take the garbage out or interact with my worn-out partner.

I have no doubt my father was a dedicated, attentive, and meticulous physician. His work also provided an escape from my mother, a Rosedale Special, who could be manipulative, demanding, even tyrannical. In the hospital, he could enact a role of "people person," free from the emotional threats of close relationships.

I'm also surprised at how much my father's colleagues know about me. Several of them, strangers to me, speak warmly of the pride my father took in my accomplishments. He clearly spoke about me at length at work.

Their remarks trigger a surge of disappointment and anger. Why the hell couldn't he express that pride and affection directly to me?

My siblings depart, and I linger in Calgary for a few days to help my mother begin the task of settling my father's affairs, many of which require a copy of his death certificate. When it arrives, it's strange to see my father's identity reduced to a few check boxes about gender, race, age, and marital status on a one-page form.

Even stranger is the primary cause of death: "Combined Overdose of Prescriped [sic] Medication (Opiates and Benzodiazepines)." What about his cancer? It's marked off as a secondary condition, contributing to death but "not causally related to the immediate cause." I flick the paper in astonishment. How ridiculous. How could my father's cancer not be causally related to his death? Without cancer, he wouldn't have been using painkillers and sedatives.

And the diagnosis of "overdose" carries an ominous overtone of negligence, even deliberation. My mother's schoolgirl grimace suddenly takes on new significance. Did she deliberately hasten his death? Does she harbour guilt? Will there be repercussions – an investigation, charges? As the days go by, no police officer arrives at the door. In the aftermath of my father's death, her lupus flares, so I don't bring the subject up.

After I return home and begin to resume a normal routine, a question simmers: How did the medical examiner arrive at the conclusion of "overdose"? In the privacy of my hospital office, I examine the form again. In one box, there's a scrawled note about the finding of "a large number of medicines available in the home." I'm not surprised: my mother possessed a hoard of painkillers and tranquilizers that she used to keep the lupus at bay. But the mere presence of medicines does not prove my father took them.

I decide to investigate. But if I enquire as mere Charles Hayter I may encounter a bureaucratic stonewall. Time to borrow my mother's strategy and switch on my own inner Rosedale Special. I pick up the microphone of my dictation machine and dictate a letter to the chief medical examiner of the Office of the Attorney General, Province of Alberta:

Dear Sir:
RE: CASE #48692 RUSSELL HAYTER DOD MAY 14/1992
I would very much like to know the evidence for stating that an overdose of medication was the cause of death. Was the level of Opiate and Benzodiazepine in my father's blood measured, and, if so, what were the levels?
Charles Hayter, MD, FRCPC

With her customary discretion, my admin assistant types this up on official letterhead and mails it off. I'm surprised when I receive a response within in a few days. The reply includes a copy of my father's toxicology report with the results of blood tests done as part of his autopsy. An invoice for $15.00 is attached.

My father's blood contained very high levels of morphine and the sedatives ("tranquilizers") lorazepam and diazepam, commonly known by their trade names: Ativan and Valium. The report has a guide to the expected "therapeutic" levels of these drugs. The amounts in my father's blood far exceeded these levels and were in the range where death from profound depression of the nervous system would occur.

To someone such as me who has spent years trying – not always successfully – to ease the pain of terminally ill cancer patients, this concept

of "therapeutic levels" is absurd. The implication is that there must somehow be a standard dose of morphine, like there is for penicillin or in-
sulin, that produces a blood level that in turn gives a standard clinical
response. But pain is not like bacterial counts or blood sugar: it's highly
subjective and escapes easy measurement. The dose of morphine suitable
for one patient might not help another. There just is no standard dose
of morphine in the context of a dying cancer patient. To achieve pain
control, the dose of narcotics must be carefully titrated to an individual
patient's pain level and side effects. Some patients tolerate large doses,
others get toxicity with only small amounts. The concept of "overdose"
is irrelevant.

Surely the chief medical examiner of Alberta knows this – but considering the ignorance of many doctors about the management of cancer
pain, maybe not. Would they want their own pain control constrained
by an arbitrary lab measurement? "I'm sorry, sir, even though you're in
terrible pain, we can't give you any more morphine, as the level in your
blood has exceeded the 'therapeutic level.'"

The medical profession's conservative attitude to pain control has often infuriated me. Time and time again, I've seen terminally ill cancer
patients in excruciating pain because their doctors or families resist the
idea of putting them on strong painkillers such as morphine. Typical
reasons include the fear of addiction – irrelevant in the context of someone who is not using the drugs for pleasure and who has limited life
expectancy – and the bizarre idea that pain is a normal part of the end of
life. Death should involve suffering, stoicism, maybe even penance. I've
also commonly encountered the idea to keep strong painkillers in reserve
for when they are "really needed" – as if that isn't *now*, when the patient
writhes and screams from the tormenting animal in the bed.

A truth remains: my father had deadly amounts of drugs in his body
when he died. Perhaps my mother did kill him, in the strictest definition
of the word. Yes, her slapdash use of "dollops" of morphine likely contributed to his death. But what quality of life did my father have to look
forward to? Bed bound, wracked with pain, dependent on others for even

the most trivial of personal care, with no hope of recovery – if such an existence was cut short by a few days or even a week, so what? That extra dollop spared him days of suffering.

As the days go by, a more unpleasant thought bubbles to the surface. Was there malice? Was that dollop in the Tang my mother's final act of vengeance? She was worn out from enacting the role of Nurse, caring for my father single-handedly. In that state of exhaustion, did her barely concealed rage at his lifelong emotional unavailability and suppression of her needs in favour of his career take over?

On that final day, as she stood in her Calgary kitchen with Trixie nuzzling at her ankles, and swirled the morphine into the sunshine-tinted glass of Tang, did her nurse's power collude with a lifetime of resentment to put an end to their mutual suffering?

I'll never know. After my father's death, my mother spirals into a vortex of depression that culminates in a suicide attempt. I find myself on another early morning flight to Calgary and making another trip to the hospital. I spend a week at her bedside and watch her ascend from the depths of comatose incoherence to a hopped-up caricature of her volatile self. After she's safely placed in a geriatric psychiatry unit, I escape home.

After her discharge, she decides to move back to England, where she spends the rest of her days as yet another of those lonely white-haired widows you spot wandering the promenades of the south coast, clinging to faint memories and shattered hopes from some long-ago life. I never discover the role of guilt over my father's death in her final depression.

In my office, I slide the folder containing my father's autopsy report into the back of a filing cabinet and push the drawer shut firmly. It's time to get on with my life.

Death stirs from the print on the wall and flutters to my red-leather recliner. His ruby eyes glint from beneath his cowl. He smiles at me.

"Think you can forget about me so easily?"

"I don't know what you mean."

"You're a smart fellow. I'll let you figure it out."

He vanishes, leaving his signature sulphurous odour.

"Wait. What are you – ?"

But he's gone.

Then it hits me.

Of course. My father's dead. I'm his eldest child.

I'm next in line.

"It makes everything so pointless." My father's anguished cry echoes through my mind.

I don't want my life to end like that. I don't want my life to be pointless.

Am I truly living the life I want to live?

I know what I have to do. I have to deal with my own deep-seated cancer.

Like many gay men of my generation and before, I hadn't dealt with my own sexuality. Just as I'd witnessed my colleagues, patients, and myself do with cancer, I'd dealt with it by hiding, refusing, denying, obfuscating, covering, deflecting. Like an ignored cancer, it continued to grow, smoulder, fester, and rob me of energy needed to live a full life.

It was time to focus some rays of healing on that cancer.

Epilogue: The Authentic Doctor

Within a few years of my father's death, I made some major life changes. I separated from my wife of twenty-two years and began the process of coming out as a gay man. I moved to Toronto to be part of the city's thriving gay community and its cultural opportunities. During my full-time medical career, I had satisfied my humanities instincts through research and writing about the history of medicine. In Toronto, I allowed my love of theatre to resurface. I dabbled in drag and did a turn as Peggy Lee in a drag revue to benefit Casey House, an AIDS hospice. I wrote and performed a one-person show, *Lady-in-Waiting*, about a doctor with a secret life as a drag queen, which picked up a writing award at a queer theatre festival in New York. Eventually, I shifted my radiation oncology schedule to part-time so I could devote more time and energy to writing. Painful as many of these steps were to those around me, they were necessary parts of my quest to avoid ending up like my father, sobbing "it makes everything so pointless" on my deathbed.

His outburst remained a vivid and perplexing memory. Outwardly, my father had lived a life that seemed far from pointless. He'd scored many "points": his schoolboy athletic trophies, his medical degree, his specialist certification, his successful career as a physiatrist, his lectures and papers, his three children, not to mention his lifelong loyalty to my irascible mother.

What exactly had he meant? Maybe he was thinking of how his professional aspirations had robbed him of time and energy for connection with his family, including his eldest son. Back in England, my mother had wanted him to settle into the life of a GP so they could enjoy a cosy domestic life. Instead, he chose a career that involved a strenuous struggle up the ladder of specialty training. What was the point of all that striving in the face of his neglect of his family? If it left him with a son that thought of him as an "old bastard"?

Maybe he was also thinking of all the psychic energy expended in concealing family secrets such as his racial origins and the separation of his parents. Again, what was the point of all that veiling and vigilance?

There were clues to other reasons in material I discovered after his death. I found a sheaf of letters in his files that bore witness to angry disputes with his hospital superiors and colleagues, disputes of which I previously had only dim awareness. My father had a suspicious and testy side, but the vehemence of these letters shocked me. He felt he had been ousted from his posts in Winnipeg and Calgary. Maybe on his deathbed he recognized the pointlessness of all that conflict.

Most surprising, there was a faded blue notebook containing poems he had written as a young man. As I read the verses, written in blue-black ink in his characteristic tiny, neat script, I wondered, did he regret not pursuing poetry further? Perhaps he had lived his life with unfulfilled creative yearnings that he never shared with his family. As a writer, I felt sad at the missed opportunity for connection through writing.

What made him shut down that side of himself? What held him back from living a truer, fuller, richer life? Throughout this book I've referred to the protocols or scripts that doctors learn and use to manage their patients – scripts that leave no room for the unpredictable, illogical, or irrational grenades hurled by patients. My father's denial of himself points to another layer of protocol, the life script for doctoring. My father followed the protocol of countless doctors before and after him: he prepared for medical school by studying science, worked hard to obtain a medical degree, then even harder to obtain his specialist qualification, and finally entered a medical world that was ruthlessly competitive. As they do to this day, newly graduated specialists vied with each other for coveted consultancy jobs, and once ensconced, competed for promotion through endless cycles of grants and publications. In the loftiest of academic hospitals, patients were nuisances whose care interfered with academic projects. Their only use was fodder for research trials. There was no space for poetry in this grim, unidimensional world. Male-dominated, the only respectable outlet was sports.

The products of this traditional script are doctors who are technically competent to treat disease but deficient in what is colloquially called bedside manner; skilled in the science of medicine but not its art. Much has been written about the art of medicine, but I'm never quite sure exactly what it means. Like the distinction between allopathic and alternative remedies, separating the art and science of medicine creates a false dichotomy. All of medicine can be thought of as an art. As my mentor, the opera-loving fashionista Dr. Vera Kraus, never failed to remind me as she brandished her red crayon over an X-ray, there is as much art in crafting a radiation volume as in breaking bad news.

The traditional script produces doctors who are artful at managing disease but not necessarily its accompanying emotional and spiritual suffering. This deficiency was recognized as long ago as the 1980s, when Dr. Raymond Bush, then director of the Ontario Cancer Institute, warned against the lure of technology in radiation oncology that distracted oncologists from seeing their patients as human beings. Riffing off the title of Izaak Walton's 1653 *The Compleat Angler*, he encouraged radiation oncologists to be "compleat oncologists," well-rounded doctors expert both in radiation technique and in the overall care and support of cancer patients, including their emotional needs. This message continues to be relevant in the twenty-first century, when the siren call of technology is ever louder in all medical specialties.

I know from experience that many doctors are content to focus on the technical aspects of care and foist the distress of a patient or family member off on a nurse or social worker, thus avoiding being drawn into complex emotional dramas. I've been tempted to do the same in the middle of a busy clinic. Such behaviour feeds the public image of doctors as cold and arrogant, one factor behind the common pursuit of alternative remedies from practitioners who are seen as more patient and compassionate than allopathic doctors. More profoundly, it diminishes our role as healers.

Thanks to the pleas of outliers such as Dr. Bush, in recent decades much has been done to rewrite the classic doctoring scenario of my father's day, beginning with new approaches to who gets cast in the role of medical student. The change in admission criteria that enabled my own entrance into medicine was meant to facilitate the entry to medical school of more rounded individuals, who, it was hoped, might be expected to become more caring, sensitive physicians than those who had just taken the science prerequisites. For many years, I was involved in the audition of candidates at a leading Canadian medical school where personal attributes were given the same weight as grades in deciding admission. On paper, it was hard to distinguish one overenthusiastically altruistic candidate from another. The final step was an in-person audition: an interview intended to assess directly interpersonal skills. If I'd asked any of these candidates whether or not they wanted to be a "compleat physician," they would have answered with an enthusiastic yes.

Once cast, medical students sometimes rehearse the emotional scenarios of their future patients. My own undergraduate training back in the early 1980s included a course called Psychosocial Aspects of Medicine (PAM), a grab bag of topics ranging from grief to sexuality. Many of my fellow students regarded it with scepticism, of uncertain value to their future careers, and skipped it entirely. Of an evening, when faced with reading an article for PAM or cracking open my pathology tome to bone up on some obscure disease, the pathology tome took precedence.

Other changes include projects such as the CanMEDS project of the Royal College of Physicians and Surgeons of Canada, which attempts to replace the old Hero model of doctoring with a more nuanced, multidimensional role that recognizes doctors as part of a team.

Within oncology, there has been an emphasis on the emotional care of patients. Large cancer centres now have departments of "supportive care" or "psychosocial oncology" with dedicated teams of specialist nurses, physicians, social workers, and psychologists intended to give patients a firmer footing on the stage and to coach them through their journey. The latest buzzword is "distress," a catch-all term for emotional responses to cancer. Many cancer centres now routinely screen new patients for distress, often with a self-administered form on which patients rate the intensity of feelings such as anxiety or depression.

Despite these measures, why do doctors' performances continue to stumble? Why do they continue to ignore or sideline patients' emotional needs? Why is the concept of the "compleat" physician still so elusive? As recently as December 2020, the *Canadian Medical Association Journal* featured an essay in which a patient received a cancer diagnosis in a busy hospital hallway. In keeping with the grand tradition of obfuscation, the doctor used the term "neoplastic" to describe the patient's illness.

I have first-hand experience of the persistent deficiencies in "bedside manner." Twice in my life I've exchanged my white coat for a blue gown and observed the theatre of medicine from a hospital bed. On both occasions, the technical aspects of my care were excellent but emotional engagement was lacking. The most noticeable defect was failure to make eye contact. One surgical resident's eyes scanned the pages of my chart the whole time she was talking to me. An intern rushed in and out of my room to place an IV line without introducing himself. His eyes remained rivetted in Dracula-like fascination on my veins. Worse yet were doctors who looked at me without seeing, faces blank masks, eyes cold, like they were inspecting a pathological specimen. Knowing I was a fellow doctor made no difference.

The abruptness of most of my caregivers made real connection startling. One morning, a surgeon plopped himself down on the side of my bed like an oversized puppy and didn't mind looking me warmly in the eyes while giving me his morning bulletin about my condition. His openness and warmth made me feel like a human being rather than a specimen. His manner engendered trust, surely the foundation of any therapeutic relationship.

What accounts for doctors' continued failure to meet the standards of empathy outlined in their training and endorsed by professional bodies? I can only offer some conjectures. Partly, it's the work environment into which they emerge from training. The root of the word "hospital" is the Latin *hospitale*, hospitable, but today's hospitals are often inhospitable "healthcare centres" run on efficiency, not compassion. Oncologists often bear the brunt of ruthless efficiency that focuses on such metrics as annual targets for patient numbers and timeliness of appointments. Quite rightly, management teams want all new cancer cases to be seen as soon as possible after referral: Who wants to keep a newly diagnosed cancer patient waiting for an appointment? But as new cancer cases inexorably rise, and the number of oncologists remains static or rises only slowly, oncologists are forced to see more patients within an appropriate time. Throughout my career, there was always pressure to see more and more patients and find creative ways of freeing up time to do so. Sometimes things got so busy I forgot the details of a patient I'd seen a few days earlier when questioned by a nurse. In this frantic environment, the first thing to go is psychosocial care. Oncologists weave from room to room, barely keeping their heads above water, clinging to their management protocols like life rafts, leaving the nurses and social workers to mop up the emotional debris.

The method of doctor evaluation is another factor. The focus in all of my annual performance reviews was on meeting my targets for case numbers, and in academic centres, my numbers of publications or presentations. Never once was a patient asked to contribute to my review; never once was my compassion or empathy assessed. Sure, there were questions about "interpersonal relationships" on the evaluation form, usually ticked off in a cursory manner by my chief. I don't know of a single hospital where performance evaluations of nurses, doctors, or technicians genuinely take into account the experience of patients. Unless there is a serious complaint of, say, abusive behaviour, a physician's interpersonal skills with patients are never closely assessed.

There's also another factor: avoidance of emotional engagement as a protective device. A 2018 study by the Canadian Medical Association found that 30 per cent of Canadian physicians experience burnout, defined as emotional exhaustion accompanied by detachment, cynicism, and reduced sense of accomplishment. A career in healthcare brings relentless contact with pain, suffering, and death, and accompanying feelings of sadness and anxiety. Medical schools and professional organizations recognize the problem and offer programs in "physician wellness" and "self-care," but most of these programs require physicians to diagnose themselves and self-refer. For many physicians, especially men, seeking help might be perceived as a sign of weakness, and the easiest path is to retreat behind a mask of cold detachment.

Finally, detachment is exacerbated by remuneration scales that reward procedures over comfort. Most specialist physicians are paid their "big bucks" for procedures, not for talking to or supporting patients. According to the current scale in Ontario for radiation oncology, the fee for counselling patients – sitting with them, explaining things, answering questions, basically offering comfort – for twenty minutes is only one-third of the fee for reviewing and approving the simplest of radiation plans. In twenty minutes, an experienced radiation oncologist can review two or more such plans. More complex radiation plans take longer, but the associated fees are higher. The fee for even an initial visit, when the focus should be on explanation and discussion, is only 70 per cent of that for a basic radiation plan. Thus, there's absolutely no financial incentive to spend time with patients. Why waste your time talking to patients and getting drawn into their emotional dramas, when you can sit in your office and earn money by fiddling with radiation plans with your computer mouse? In truth, the incentive is to nudge your patients towards having radiation and getting the fee for planning. Even in a free-market model, procedures are more lucrative than direct patient contact.

I worry that the formalization of distress assessment only adds another step to the management protocols and just encourages the mindset that oncology can be reduced to a script. Distress assessment ticked, right, let's move to the next step. Worst of all, screening forms and reflexive referrals to social work abrogate oncologists of their responsibilities to care for patients' emotional well-being. To put it another way, it leads us further away from, not towards, Bush's notion of the "compleat oncologist."

One caveat: much of what I'm discussing refers only to specialist medicine, the medicine practised behind the walls of hospitals that focuses on procedures such as surgery or radiotherapy and in which I have the most experience. Family doctors in community offices are likely free from the pressures of efficiency and the vigilance of the bureaucracy of hospitals and are able to offer patients more time and empathy. This is true of my own family doctor. He doesn't mind just sitting with me and chatting. I suspect there's method to his behaviour: while we chat, I notice him assessing nuances of my body language and inflection.

I don't have a magic bullet for the problem of the Detached Doctor, but my father's *cri de coeur* holds an important clue. His rigid adherence to a script for his life held him back from living a true, authentic life, one in which he might have unburdened himself of secrets, allowed himself to write poetry, and generally experienced more joy. What kind of person would he then have become? More germane, what kind of doctor would he have been?

An encounter with a patient involves science, art – and authenticity. I don't want to belabour the coming-out metaphor, but the closet is an apt image for so much of what happens in medicine. Doctors conduct case conferences behind closed doors; they are reluctant to discuss taboo subjects such as sexuality, treatment failure, or death; and they hide their feelings behind professional masks. I would argue that doctors only truly connect with patients when they allow themselves the freedom to step from the closet, loosen their professional masks, and let their authentic selves shine. The traditional script makes this almost impossible:

doctors are not supposed to be vulnerable, display emotion, or become attached to patients. Even a slight opening of the closet door brings huge self-flagellation, which only adds to stress and greater concealment. Like my father, most doctors are incredibly hard on themselves in their attempts to measure up.

Yet the truth is, we are as human as our patients. Authenticity involves revealing our humanity, admitting our failures, and also developing self-compassion. As self-compassion emerges, so does greater compassion for our patients.

I have first-hand experience of this phenomenon. After my separation from my wife, I was wracked with doubt and guilt over a decision that had inflicted enormous pain on her and her family. At the urging of a friend, I attended a gay men's spiritual retreat at a centre in the wooded hills of Pennsylvania. There I met many men with life journeys similar to my own, men who had lifelong struggles with their sexuality within heterosexual marriages. Through my conversations and reflections there, I began to feel a glimmer of compassion towards myself.

When I went back to work the following week and started seeing patients again, I was surprised to find stronger compassion for them welling up inside me. I had always considered myself to be a compassionate doctor, willing and able to connect with my patients the way I'd seen Dr. Friar do, but I suddenly found my patients' stories touched me in a deeper way than ever before. At the bedside of one man dying of prostate cancer, my eyes unexpectedly brimmed with tears. He responded with tears of his own.

Not all doctors will have life-altering experiences such as coming out that plant within them the seed of compassion. Galloping breathlessly on the frantic treadmill of modern medical practice, how can a doctor achieve authenticity?

The answer is in front of us: our patients. As Vera Peters said, "You learn more from the patient than you do from the books."

Throughout my career, strangers often reacted with horror when I told them I'm an oncologist. "How can you spend your life dealing with cancer and death?" they asked, sometimes unconsciously recoiling, as if I harboured the contagion of cancer. I often asked myself the same question: What keeps me going in this gruesome business of cancer?

It took me a long time to see that I drew strength not from any mystical inner power but from my patients and their willingness to be authentic with me.

I think of

the jubilation of Betty, which restored my confidence;
the stoicism and humour of Christie, which disarmed my fear;
the wisdom of Sam and George, which cut through my obfuscation;
the obstinacy of Peter, which made me see my own hubris;
the desperation of Cindy and Jim, which gave me resolve;
the gratitude of Lori, which brought me cheer;
the grace of Tom, which helped to heal my guilt;
the unspoken kindness of Mr. Singh, which soothed my anxiety;
even the anger of Justice McNichol and Sandra, which opened
    compassion through a glimpse of their pain; and
finally, my father's angst, which opened the path to my own
    authenticity.

These patients, and countless others, were courageous enough to open themselves to me. Actually, they had little choice. Unlike doctors, patients have no script. Like a nervous understudy called on to cover a major role at the last minute, a cancer patient is suddenly thrust on a stage. The summons is immediate, insistent, cruel. They stumble from the wings naked and bewildered, blinded by the bright lights, trying desperately to find their marks. Emotions can erupt in torrents more like operatic arias than ballads.

If patients can do it for us, then why can't we do it for them?

It's helpful to remember the ancestry doctors share with actors. Both trace their origin to the shaman or medicine person of many cultures. The shaman effected healing through masks, costumes, props, dances, songs, and rituals, and most of all, a healing presence, like that of my professor in my summer internship. One of the paradoxes of acting is that the most believable, effective acting does not come from pretending, from faking emotions, but from the actor's ability to delve deep inside to find and present emotional truth – in other words, to be authentic. Authenticity has power both on the stage and in the consulting room.

For their part, patients should not let doctors get away with anything less. They should not tolerate the behaviour of hand-puppet oncologists who pop their heads around the door for a quick hello or keep their eyes glued to the chart during a conversation. Of course, doctors know damn well they can get away with this because patients are vulnerable and unlikely to complain out of fear of a backlash. That's why hospitals and other institutions need to develop better processes for assessment of physicians' behaviour. Perhaps patients should be asked about distress caused by physicians – "iatrogenic distress" – in addition to that caused by illness.

The payoffs are potentially huge: less stress and burnout, more satisfaction with work, greater compliance on the part of patients with treatment, and ultimately more joy in work. How much more interesting and joyful is it to see the woman before us as a fully rounded human than just another case of T3 breast cancer? How much more joyful and rich would medical practice be if we allowed ourselves to go off script – to share details of our personal lives, make self-deprecating jokes, laugh, touch, and cry with our patients?

All doctors can find such opportunities for moments of real connection with their patients.

If they can't, they need to ask why. I suspect it's fear that holds them back. The greatest fear is of Death, that dark, stalking figure whose presence is summoned by staring into a cancer patient's face. Even if the patient is, as many are, curable, cancer holds Death in such a tight embrace of mental association that the two entities are difficult to separate. Simply put, every cancer patient is a reminder of our own mortality who brings into focus uncomfortable questions about the pointlessness of our lives.

As fear dissolves and the mask slips away, we can, we must find connection with a fellow human being on the same journey with the same end. The only difference between us is that for the patient, the end has become real.

Acknowledgments

This book would not have come to fruition without the help and encouragement of many individuals.

My biggest debt of gratitude is to my former patients, whose situations provided inspiration for my characters and stories. As a mentor once told me, medicine allows a unique window into the lives of other human beings, and I am grateful to have been given that opportunity.

My siblings Robert Hayter and Sally Brown, and my children Rosie Parris and Jonathan Hayter, shared memories of my father's illness and death that helped me to reconstruct his story.

In the book's creation, I owe particular thanks to Susan Olding, my writing coach, who introduced me to the pleasures of creative non-fiction and gave helpful feedback on early drafts of many of the chapters. I also recognize my fellow scribes Alison Li and Marianne Fedunkiw for their friendship, encouragement, and advice during the writing and editing process.

Kimberly de Witte and the members of her West End Writers Group gave feedback on early drafts over coffee and treats during morning meetings at Baka Bakery Café on Bloor Street West. Similarly, Jeff Joachim Schmidt and members of his Writers' Connector group provided helpful feedback during Sunday evening gatherings at Jeff's cosy apartment.

I am grateful to Dr. T. "Jock" Murray and my ex-colleagues Dr. Judith Balogh and Dr. Ida Ackerman for their expert review and helpful comments on the entire manuscript.

My partner Mark Tan contributed comfort, nourishment, and advice during the several cycles of drafts and redrafts. Others who provided help along the way include Beth Kaplan, Dr. Teresa Nelson, Dr. Jonathan Tsao, Janet Joy Wilson, and Dr. Camilla Zimmermann. I was delighted when my former theatre professor, Richard Trousdell, reviewed the introductory chapter.

Finally, I would like to acknowledge the support and encouragement of the staff of UTP, particularly my editor, Meg Patterson, who helped shape an amorphous collection of stories into a cohesive narrative and also gave me the nudge I needed to weave the story of my father's illness through the whole book. I am grateful as well to Catherine Plear for her eagle-eyed copy-editing of the final manuscript.